THE CAROTID AND THE EYE

Edited by

Ramon Berguer, M.D., Ph.D.
Harold Weiss, M.D., F.A.C.S.

PRAEGER

PRAEGER SPECIAL STUDIES • PRAEGER SCIENTIFIC

New York • Philadelphia • Eastbourne, UK
Toronto • Hong Kong • Tokyo • Sydney

Library of Congress Cataloging in Publication Data
Main entry under title:
The Carotid and the eye.
Evolved from an interdisciplinary conference held in Detroit, Mich. in Apr. 1984.
Includes index.
1. Retina—Blood-vessels—Diseases—Congresses. 2. Carotid artery—Diseases—Complications and sequelae—Congresses. 3. Eye—Blood-vessels—Diseases—Congresses. I. Berguer, Ramon. II. Weiss, Harold, 1941- . [DNLM: 1. Carotid Artery Diseases—complications—congresses. 2. Eye—blood supply—congresses. 3. Eye Diseases—etiology—congresses. 4. Retinal Artery—congresses. 5. Retinal Diseases—complications—congresses. WW 140 C293 1984]
RE661.V3C37 1985 617.7′3 85-6336
ISBN 0-03-000043-2 (alk. paper)

Published in 1985 by Praeger Publishers
CBS Educational and Professional Publishing, a Division of CBS Inc.
521 Fifth Avenue, New York, NY 10175 USA

56789 052 987654321

Printed in the United States of America on acid-free paper

INTERNATIONAL OFFICES

Orders from outside the United States should be sent to the appropriate address listed below. Orders from areas not listed below should be placed through CBS International Publishing, 383 Madison Ave., New York, NY 10175 USA

Australia, New Zealand
Holt Saunders, Pty, Ltd., 9 Waltham St., Artarmon, N.S.W. 2064, Sydney, Australia

Canada
Holt, Rinehart & Winston of Canada, 55 Horner Ave., Toronto, Ontario, Canada M8Z 4X6

Europe, the Middle East, & Africa
Holt Saunders, Ltd., 1 St. Anne's Road, Eastbourne, East Sussex, England BN21 3UN

Japan
Holt Saunders, Ltd., Ichibancho Central Building, 22-1 Ichibancho, 3rd Floor, Chiyodaku, Tokyo, Japan

Hong Kong, Southeast Asia
Holt Saunders Asia, Ltd., 10 Fl, Intercontinental Plaza, 94 Granville Road, Tsim Sha Tsui East, Kowloon, Hong Kong

Manuscript submissions should be sent to the Editorial Director, Praeger Publishers, 521 Fifth Avenue, New York, NY 10175 USA

THE CAROTID AND THE EYE

LIST OF CONTRIBUTORS

Ramon Berguer, M.D., Ph.D.
Professor of Surgery, Wayne State University and
Chief, Section of Vascular Surgery, Harper-Grace Hospitals
Department of Surgery
6-C University Health Center
4201 St. Antoine
Detroit, MI 48201

A. Joel Feldman, M.D.
8402 Harcourt Road
Suite 500
Indianapolis, IN 46260

Anton N. Hasso, M.D.
Associate Professor of Radiology and
Chief of the Section of Neuroradiology
Loma Linda University
School of Medicine
Loma Linda, CA 92350

Sohan S. Hayreh, M.D., Ph.D.
Professor of Ophthalmology
The University of Iowa Hospitals and Clinics
Department of Ophthalmology
Iowa City, IA 52242

Paul Henkind, M.D., Ph.D.
Professor and Chairman
Department of Ophthalmology
Albert Einstein College of Medicine of Yeshiva University
Montefiore Hospital and Medical Center
111 East 210th Street
Bronx, NY 10467

Roger F. Higgins, Ph.D.
Director, Vascular Surgery Laboratory
Harper-Grace Hospitals
3990 John R
Detroit, MI 48201

Robert S. Jampel, M.D., Ph.D.
Professor and Chairman
Department of Ophthalmology
The Kresge Eye Institute of Wayne State University
3994 John R
Detroit, MI 48201

Edouard Kieffer, M.D.
Professeur Agrege à la Faculté de Medicine de Paris
Chirurgien des Hospitaux de Paris
Service de Chirurgie Vasculaire
Groupe Hospitalier Pitié-Salpétrière
83, Boulevard de 1 'Hôpital
75651 PARIS Cedex 13 FRANCE

Alfredo Lazo, M.D.
Department of Radiology
Harper-Grace Hospitals
3990 John R
Detroit, MI 48201

Larry E. Magargal, M.D.
Co-Director Retina Vascular Unit
Willis Eye Hospital
9th & Walnut St.
Philadelphia, PA 19107

Charles G. Rob, M.D.
Professor of Surgery
Uniformed Services University of the Health Sciences
School of Medicine
4301 Jones Bridge Road
Bethesda, MD 20814

R.W. Ross Russell, M.D.
Department of Neurology
St. Thomas' Hospital
London, SE1 7EH ENGLAND

Robert G. Siekert, M.D.
Department of Neurology
Mayo Clinic
Rochester, MN 55905

Alexander J. Walt, M.D., Ch.B.
Professor and Chairman
Department of Surgery
Wayne State University
School of Medicine
6-C University Health Center
4201 St. Antoine
Detroit, MI 48201

Edward A. Waybright, M.D.
Assistant Professor
Department of Neurology
Division of Neuro-Ophthalmology
Medical College of Virginia
Box 559 MCV Station
Richmond, VA 23298

Harold Weiss, M.D., F.A.C.S.
Assistant Professor of Ophthalmology
Kresge Eye Institute, Wayne State University and Retina Consultants of Michigan
29201 Telegraph Road
Southfield, MI 48034

David M. Worthen, M.D.
Assistant Chief, Medical Director for Academic Affairs
Office of Academic Affairs (14)
Veterans Administration
810 Vermont Ave. N.W.
Washington, DC 20420

Brian R. Younge, M.D.
Associate Professor of Ophthalmology
Department of Ophthalmology
Mayo Clinic
Rochester, MN 55905

PREFACE

This book evolved from an interdisciplinary conference held in Detroit, Michigan in April, 1984. The conference brought together participants from related but different specialties to address problems which are common to all, but seldom discussed in an interdisciplinary manner. The conference was the result of ten years of personal and professional collaboration in our work at the Kresge Eye Institute and the Division of Vascular Surgery at Wayne State University/Harper-Grace Hospitals.

The anatomy and pathology of the orbital vasculature comprise a very thin slice of medical knowledge. There is little factual information about this body cavity: its contents are not accessible to direct inspection and are poorly displayed by new techniques such as CT scanning or selective arteriography. Furthermore social tradition has generally proscribed postmortem investigations of the orbit and consequently we have meager knowledge of the intrinsic pathology of the vessels that supply the retina or the optic nerve.

From the ophthalmologist's point of view, the problems needing extradisciplinary expertise involved central retinal artery occlusions, branch artery occlusions, central retinal vein occlusions, amaurosis fugax, scintillating scotomata and hypoperfusion oculopathy. There was also a growing sense that ischemic optic neuropathy is, to some degree, associated with occlusive disease of the carotid system. From the vascular surgeon's viewpoint, there was the need for evaluation of the patients who were found to have ocular symptoms or signs either prior to or subsequent to carotid or vertebral operations. What evolved over the years was a working relationship in which ophthalmologists and vascular surgeons began to think and approach problems in accord. Through this cooperation we realized how much each could contribute to the other's understanding and treatment of the problems seen.

This volume is the first attempt to bridge gaps in our understanding of orbital problems, perhaps a consequence of our specialization. We hope that it will stimulate further cooperation among ophthalmologists, vascular surgeons, neuroradiologists and neurologists. Our discussions have raised a new set of questions that need to be answered. We look forward to other efforts to clarify them.

Ramon Berguer
Harold Weiss

CONTENTS

THE CAROTID AND THE EYE

INTRODUCTION

THE CAROTID AND THE EYE: THEIR HISTORICAL CONNECTION

Alexander J. Walt, M.D.

My friend and colleague, Dr. Ramon Berguer, has an exquisite sense of irony. He invited me to fly in from the American Surgical Association meeting to attend the symposium on the carotid and the eye. The role of Chairman as a Visiting Professor to his own department has frequently been advanced in jest; I believe this is the first time it has, in fact, become a reality. Undoubtedly, it will not be the last time I shall hear about this phenomenon.

My topic was selected for me by Dr. Berguer because we run a weekly series of historical vignettes in our Department of Surgery. These presentations are usually given by one of our medical students. Dr. Berguer thought it would perhaps be instructive for me to reflect on the historical evolution of how we came to appreciate that the carotid and the eye are married for better or for worse, in sickness and in health, until death do they part. When I went to the literature, I immediately had a sense of nostalgia because so many who have contributed to this field were at the Mayo Clinic while I was a resident there. As so often happens, I completely failed to appreciate the great flowering of this field in the institution at that time. The names of the staff then constitute a roll call of the great contributors—Millikan; Siekert (who is here today); Kearns, who wrote a superb account of the historical development of this field; Hollenhorst, who gave his name to a clinical phenomenon; and Whisnant, who was a resident with me. About the same time, in our own institution, Wayne State University, Dr. John E. Webster and Dr. Steve Gurdjian were also doing pioneering surgical surgery in this field.

The main value of developing a historical perspective is the stimulus it gives to research and the acquisition of salutary humility that it allows. The exercise also reminds one that there must be vital phenomena currently being ignored just as certainly as we previously ignored the association between carotid disease and ocular signs and symptoms for so long. Our blindness to events that stare at us is often monumental, and the amount of time that elapses between solid observations and the correct interpretation of these is always intriguing. Amaurosis fugax was so named in 1922 by Moore (1). In 1947 when I was a medical student using Walsh's textbook (2), this entity was still said to be due to spasm of the retinal artery and to be benign. Most ophthalmologists, surgeons and others were until the last decade blind to the warning signals - and some still are. The question is why? Probably for reasons of communication or, more properly stated perhaps, noncommunication. When strokes subsequently occurred in patients who had previously had premonitory eye signs attended to by an ophthalmologist or family physician, the immediate catastrophic event was usually treated by an internist or neurologist without knowledge of the earlier symptoms and consequently without the necessary in-depth view of the clinical problem.

The second point is really one of selective neglect. Until the 1950s, clinicians were unconcerned about examining the carotids, and pathologists ignored them at autopsies. Furthermore, ophthalmologists somehow overlooked the eye signs which we now know so well. The seminal work of Miller Fisher changed all this in a series of classic papers written in the 1950s (3,4). We should, of course, have known better. No less a genius than the ubiquitous Virchow described thrombosis of the carotid artery at autopsy in 1856 in a patient with monocular blindness (5). Other famous names such as Kussmaul in 1872 (6), and Chiari in 1905 (7) made similar observations. Nevertheless, in the 57 years which followed Virchow's report of carotid occlusion, very few comments were made on carotid abnormalities. It was not until 1913 that Ramsey Hunt (8) of Columbia University noted that visual disturbance and vascular changes in the optic nerve sometimes preceded cerebral symptoms and signs.

The third factor relates to the dependence of developments in surgery—and presumably to all human endeavors—upon the availability and impact of new technology. Until the introduction of carotid angiography in 1927 by Moniz, permitting delineation of lesions in the carotids, changes in the living subject could neither be recorded nor studied objectively. In 1950, only 23 years later, Webster and Gurdjian of the Department of Surgery at Wayne State University, supported by the Kresge Research Fund which still supports our Department of Ophthalmology at Wayne State University and the Harper-Grace Hospitals, reported four cases of spontaneous thrombosis of carotid arteries in the neck (9).

It is a tragic irony that Dr. Webster, just a few years later, was to become disabled by the disease which he was studying. Interestingly, in Case One of the series, he recorded that the patient early in his history became aware of visual impairment; in Case Three, the patient complained of blurring of vision four months before his stroke developed. The implications of this, however, were not recognized in 1950. It was not until 1951 that Fisher (3), to whom so much is owed, described transient monocular blindness as a prelude to stroke and suggested that emboli from thrombotic material in the carotid artery were responsible. The following year, Wagener (10) speculated that arteriography might be justified in all cases of amaurosis fugax so that 24 years after Moniz's introduction of this technique, Wagener went on to present the first observations of cholesterol emboli in the retina. In 1955, Millikan and Siekert (11) stressed the importance of the transient visual disturbances and recognized for the first time that the ulcerated plaque is an ever-present danger. The field now moved very rapidly and in 1959, Fisher (4) described retinal platelet emboli which may produce occlusive disease. In 1961, Hollenhorst (12) in a description that can only be described as lyrical, wrote about cholesterol crystals tumbling and moving and flashing. Noting these emboli in the retinal arteries of about 15% of patients undergoing carotid endarterectomy, Hollenhorst pointed out that although these cholesterol emboli seldom produced occlusion in the eye, they were nevertheless harbingers of cerebral disaster. In the following year, Hollenhorst (13) went on to prove the nature of these phenomena experimentally by injection studies which showed that the presence of cholesterol crystals in the ocular vessels constituted evidence of a lesion downstream, something which everybody, in retrospect, should have appreciated far earlier.

In 1963, the microaneurysms, large irregular veins, venous sludging and local hemorrhages shown us so nicely by Dr. Siekert at this conference were described by Kearns and Hollenhorst (14) as the entity of so-called venous stasis angiopathy. An occasional concomitant of carotid occlusive disease and its attendant ischemia, the physiology of this complex is still not perfectly clear. The analogy between the eye and the changes of venous stasis associated with slowing of blood flow in the lower leg cannot be ignored. In the same paper, Kearns and Hollenhorst drew attention to the entity of ischemic orbital pain. Later, in 1979, they reviewed ischemic orbital pain in relation to carotid artery bypass with a consequent improvement of blood flow that relieved the pain dramatically (15). In the leg, we might call a similar phenomenon rest pain or claudication. Analogies are dangerous and, with my ignorance in this field, I shrink from pursuing these further.

The fact is that too many of us have still not learned the lessons that the eye displays for our enlightenment. At the 1984 American Board of Surgery examinations, candidates asked about the significance of the Hollenhorst plaque pleaded ignorance for the most part. Many did so with dry mouths and ashen faces and presumably all had reduced retinal artery pressures. We should be disturbed that in 1984, representatives of our training programs still remain so ignorant of what should now be a well recognized and important entity. There is obviously much work to be done in our own discipline and, I would suspect, in your disciplines too.

Finally, the whole purpose of reviewing a field is to ask where the terra incognita now lies. Has the entire vascular ocular territory been fully explored? Obviously not. Where should we look to explain the still unexplained phenomena? Are we using the newer technology available to us to its fullest extent? We have, after all, come a long way from Moniz's arteriography to the world of NMR, CT scans and immunoassays.

Above all, recognizing that we are no different from our predecessors, we need to seek the abnormalities that are staring at us right now and which we are scanning with uncomprehending eyes. We can be sure of one thing—that there are some. In retrospect, we belatedly recognized events occurring in what may be termed the front of the eye. Perhaps it is time to enlist the help of the newer techniques to probe the hidden areas behind the eye more analytically than we have done. Some very exciting mysteries must lie in the region waiting to be illuminated.

REFERENCES

1. Moore, R.F.: *Medical Ophthalmology.* Philadelphia: P. Blakiston, Son and Co, 1922, p. 63.
2. Walsh, F.B.: *Clinical Neuro-Ophthalmology.* Baltimore: Williams and Wilkins Co, 1947, p.1031.
3. Fisher, M.: Occlusion of the internal carotid artery. *Arch. Neurol. Psychiatr.* 65:346, 1951.
4. Fisher, C.M.: Observations of the fundus oculi in transient monocular blindness. *Neurology* (Minneapolis) 9:333, 1959.
5. Virchow, R.: Zur pathologischen Anatomie der Netzhaut und des Sehnerven. *Arch. Pathol. Anat. Physiol. Klin, Med.* 10:170, 1856.
6. Kussmaul, A.: Zwei Falle von spontaner allmahlicher Verschliessung grosser Halsarterienstamme. *Deutsche Klin.* 24:461, 1872.
7. Chiari, H.: Uber das Verhalten des Teilungswinkels der Carotis communis bei der Endarteriitis chronica deformans. *Verhandl. d. deutsch. path. Gesellsch.* 9:326, 1905.
8. Hunt, J.R.: The role of the carotid arteries, in the causation of vascular lesions of the brain, with remarks on certain special features of the symptomatology. *Am. J. Med. Sci.* 147:704, 1914.
9. Webster, J.E., Dolgoff, S., and Gurdjian, E.S.: Spontaneous thrombosis of the carotid arteries in the neck. Report of four cases. *Arch. Neurol. Psychiatr.* 63:942, 1950.
10. Wagener, H.P.: Amaurosis fugax. *Am. J. Med. Sci.* 224:229, 1952.
11. Millikan, C.H., and Siekert, R.G.: Studies in cerebrovascular disease. 4. The syndrome of intermittent insufficiency of the carotid arterial system. *Proc. Staff Meet. Mayo Clin.* 30:186, 1955.
12. Hollenhorst, R.W.: Significance of bright plaques in the retinal arterioles. *Trans. Am. Ophthalmol. Soc.* 59:252, 1961.
13. Hollenhorst, R.W., Lensink, E.R., and Whisnant, J.P.: Experimental embolization of the retinal arterioles. *Trans. Am. Ophthalmol. Soc.* 60:316, 1962.

14. Kearns, T.P., and Hollenhorst, R.W.: Venous-stasis retinopathy of occlusive disease of the carotid artery. *Proc. Staff Meet. Mayo Clin.* 38:304, 1963.
15. Kearns, T.P., Siekert, R.G., and Sundt, T.M., Jr.: The ocular aspects of bypass surgery of the carotid artery. *Mayo Clinic Proc.* 54:3, 1979.

I

THE CAROTID

1

SURFACE CHARACTERISTICS AND BEHAVIOR OF CAROTID PLAQUES

A. Joel Feldman, M.D.

Lesions of the carotid artery are most commonly located at its bifurcation and may become symptomatic through one of two mechanisms: (a) embolization of atheromatous or thrombotic debris into the intracranial vasculature, or (b) reduction of flow secondary to a hemodynamically significant stenosis. The overwhelming majority of these lesions are secondary to atherosclerosis with less than 1% due to fibromuscular dysplasia. Intimal hyperplasia may occur in a vessel that has undergone previous endarterectomy. The surface characteristics of a plaque are an important determinant of its tendency to embolize, and they may also affect flow directly by influencing a plaque's tendency to form thrombus on its surface and thus further reduce flow.

Of the two mechanisms, embolism or flow reduction, evidence suggests that embolism is the more important. This knowledge has stimulated an interest in the morphology of the carotid plaque from which these emboli originate. Some of the earliest and clearest evidence that emboli may originate from extracranial carotid disease comes from the work of Fisher (1) and Hollenhorst (2) describing retinal artery embolization.

REVIEW OF THE LITERATURE

In 1862 Panum (3) first described embolization of atheromatous material in the peripheral vascular system. The first description of cerebral emboli and infarction in association with a mural thrombus at the carotid bifurcation was in 1905 by Chairi (4). Flory described atheromatous emboli from an aortic arch plaque in 1945 (5). Despite this earlier work the importance of embolism as a mechanism of central nervous system ischemia was not appreciated until more recently. Fisher in 1952 described a case of monocular blindness associated with contralateral hemiplegia; in 1959 he described the retina of a patient during an episode of monocular blindness (1). He proposed that platelet fibrin emboli traversing the retinal arteries explained the findings.

Hollenhorst described brightly colored refractile plaques in the retinal arterioles of 31 of 328 patients with clinical signs and symptoms of either carotid or vertebrobasilar disease in 1961 (2). He believed these plaques to be cholesterol crystals which had embolized from proximally located atheromatous plaques. In seven patients the retinal plaques had appeared during or immediately following operation on the carotid bifurcation. David confirmed that these plaques were cholesterol using histochemical testing in 1963 (6).

Kollarits and his associates described 70 patients with retinal strokes in 1972 (7). Fifty-eight of these patients complained of amaurosis fugax, and bright plaques or platelet fibrin plugs were seen on fundoscopic examination. Fifty-three patients had no obvious source of emboli other than extracranial carotid artery disease. Forty-five underwent cerebral angiography, and carotid bifurcation plaques were identified in 43 of them (96%). Rosenthal et al described a case of sudden monocular blindness in a patient with fundoscopic evidence of central retinal artery occlusion (8). Cerebral arteriography revealed an ulcerated plaque at the carotid bifurcation which was confirmed at the time of endarterectomy. Cerebral emboli to the brain from atherosclerotic aortic arch lesions were described by Winter (9) and Sturgil (10). Gunning et al. presented a series of patients with either transient ischemic attacks or amaurosis fugax in whom platelet fibrin thrombi were found adhering to atherosclerotic plaques at the carotid bifurcation site at the time of operation (11). Wood and Carell presented a series of 160 patients with cerebral ischemia of whom 54% had ulcerated plaques diagnosed by angiography and surgery (12). Ehrenfeld and his associates presented 44 patients with amaurosis fugax and ipsilateral carotid lesions discovered at the time of surgery (13). Thus, embolism is an important cause of cerebral ischemia as well as ocular ischemia.

Moore and his associates described 35 patients who underwent carotid endarterectomy because of nonstenotic ulcerated plaques of the carotid bifurcation (14). Thirty-one of these patients had a history of transient ischemic attacks of the anterior cerebral circulation. Included were seven patients with a history of amaurosis fugax. All were cured of their symptoms for a period extending to 39 months of follow-up. Pessin et al reported on 64 patients who had experienced an acute stroke (15). All patients underwent arteriography, and 66% of these were found to have evidence of intracranial embolism distal to their extracranial carotid disease.

ANATOMICAL DESCRIPTION

The embolic material is composed of either atheromatous debris or platelet fibrin plugs originating from the surface of the carotid plaque. Thus, the surface characteristics and morphology of the plaque will determine both its tendency to embolize and the type of embolic material it generates. An understanding of the pathophysiology of an atherosclerotic plaque is important to the understanding of plaque morphology and surface characteristics.

The normal arterial wall is composed of three layers. The intima is lined on its lumenal surface by the endothelial cells. Normally a thin subendothelial layer contains scant amounts of extracellular connective tissue matrix, an occasional myointimal cell, and rare blood monocytes. Small amounts of all plasma proteins including lipoproteins are also found in the intima. The outer layer of the intima is bound by the internal elastic lamina. In the child the intima is very thin; however, with age, it thickens, accumulating ground substance and smooth muscle cells.

The media consists of large numbers of smooth muscle cells in either single or multiple layers, depending on the location. This layer also contains large numbers of collagen fibers and elastic fibers contributing strength and elasticity to the vessel wall. This same medial layer is bounded by the external elastic lamina.

The adventitia is the outermost layer of the artery and consists of smooth muscle cells, fibroblasts, collagen, and elastic fibers. It also contains the vasa vasorum which penetrate the external elastic lamina to supply the outer layers of the media (16).

ATHEROSCLEROSIS—FORMATION OF LESION

Atherosclerosis is a disease of the intima which, when severe, may involve the media and even adventitia. The earliest atheromatous lesion is probably a focal intimal accumulation of smooth muscle cells containing intracellular lipid vacuoles (foam cells). Some of these foam cells may be blood-derived monocytes. As the number of foam cells increases the early "yellow streak" or "fatty streak" lesion appears. Not all such lesions progress to atherosclerosis as they are found even in infancy in areas atypical for adult atherosclerosis. One response to this accumulation may be a progressively increased amount of collagen within the plaque which forms a fibrous or fibromuscular plaque that may impinge upon the lumen. There may be accumulation of extracellular lipids, of dead cells within the plaque, and of blood-born lipids and lipoproteins moving through the damaged endothelium. Calcification may occur within the plaque. Ulceration of the luminal surface can occur, exposing necrotic fatty debris to the lumen of the vessel. Embolization of the plaque's atheromatous content (cholesterol crystals, cholesterol esters, cellular debris) may occur.

Platelet fibrin aggregrates may also be found on the surface of such complex plaques. Atheromata have been shown to contain abnormally low amounts of prostacyclin which may predispose them to the formation of thrombus on their surface. Alternatively, thrombus may form over the irregular thrombogenic surface of an ulcerated plaque. With severe disease the media is invaded, eliciting an inflammatory response and neovascularization by the vasa vasorum. As further cell necrosis and destruction of the arterial wall occurs hemorrhage into the plaque from these vasa vasorum may occur causing a narrowing of the vessel lumen or rupture of the hemorrhagic material into the lumen. An ulcer is thus formed which may embolize or propagate thrombus locally.

ENDOTHELIAL INJURY

Current thought postulates that atherogenesis occurs as a response to continuous endothelial injury (16,17). The platelet plays an important role in this hypothesis. Platelets adhere to sites of endothelial cell injury and release platelet mitogenic factor which stimulates smooth muscle cell and fibroblast proliferation in the intima. The injury may be mechanical secondary to arterial wall vibration, direct external trauma, hypertension or shear forces. This would explain the occurrence of atherosclerotic lesions at arterial bifurcations and at areas of transition between relatively fixed and more mobile portions of the arterial tree. Any number of chemical agents are known to cause endothelial cell injury, including high serum cholesterol or lipoprotein levels, certain of the agents contained within cigarettes, homocystinemia, uremia, and certain immunological disorders. Along with proliferation of smooth muscle cells, local injury may also allow direct infiltration of plasma proteins, lipids and cells. Repeated injury, such as occurs in the situations described above, leads to the development of the atherosclerotic plaque.

PLAQUE

The morphology and surface characteristics of plaque may determine its clinical significance in a number of ways. The ulcerated plaque may expose subintimal deposits of atheromatous gruel. This gruel contains both cholesterol crystals as well as various cholesterol esters. In addition, there is a component of nonlipid debris composed of the detritus of necrotic cells. These various components have been shown to have differing thrombogenic potential when embolized into the intracranial circulation in animals (18). Thus, not only the surface characteristics of the plaque but the nature of the subintimal material exposed will determine the nature of the ischemic event that occurs. Subintimal hemorrhage may occur from ruptured vasa vasorum and cause ulceration of the plaque or sudden narrowing of the vessel lumen. Rupture or erosion of the overlying fibrous intimal cap will expose fresh thrombus (containing fibrin and platelet aggregates) to the lumen. These may embolize or propagate into the lumen, producing further impairment of flow and a source of emboli.

Ultramicroscopic ulceration and thrombi, not visible by preoperative arteriography or gross intraoperative inspection may be present and cause symptoms. Hertzer et al. examined endarterectomy specimens from ten patients (19). Eight were found to have ultramicroscopic ulceration and thrombi not appreciated by previous examination. Five patients had had transient ischemic events preoperatively.

Smooth atheromata may produce emboli by one of several mechanisms. The endothelium overlying the atheromata has been shown to contain abnormally low levels of prostacyclin predisposing it to the formation of intraluminal thrombi. It has also been postulated that the thrombogenic potential of endothelium overlying subintimal hemorrhage is enhanced and may allow thrombus formation.

Imparato and his colleagues have published the most extensive experience to date relating morphologic plaque characteristics to symptoms (20). Plaques were grouped into five major types of gross morphologic appearance. These categories were: simple plaque, ulcerated plaque, hemorrhagic plaque, lumen thrombus, and smooth plaque containing atheromatous debris. Two hundred seventy-five plaques were symptomatic and 101 were asymptomatic. Of the five plaque characteristics mentioned above, only the presence of plaque hemorrhage, present in 37% of the plaques, was statistically associated with an increased incidence of symptomatology. The most common gross morphologic characteristic was that of ulceration, present in 50% of plaques. Luzby and his group reported a very high incidence of acute or recent intraplaque hemorrhage in symptomatic patients as compared with asymptomatic patients (21). Although ulceration was commonly present in their patients, it did not correlate significantly with the presence or absence of symptoms. Interestingly, both groups reported a significant number of patients who remained symptomatic despite treatment with aspirin.

PATIENT DATA

Figure 1.1 shows the operative specimen of a patient who presented with a left hemispheric stroke manifested by a residual right hemiparesis. At

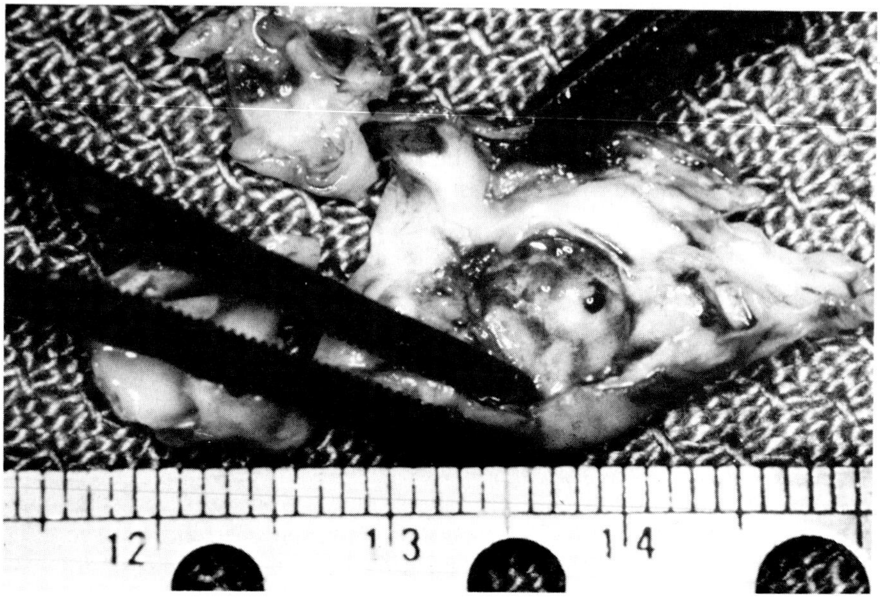

Fig. 1.1. Endarterectomy specimen showing complex plaque with large central ulceration and small amounts of fibrinous debris adherent to surface of ulceration and plaque.

the time of surgery a complex plaque with a large ulcer located centrally and small amounts of fibrin adherent to the roughened surface of the plaque were found. Figure 1.2 presents the preoperative arteriogram of a patient with a history of left hemispheric transient ischemic attacks. It reveals the classic radiologic appearance of an ulcerated plaque at the bifurcation of the carotid artery. At the time of surgery a hemorrhagic plaque which had ulcerated through the overlying endothelium with fresh thrombus contained within its base was found (Figure 1.3). An example of an asymptomatic Hollenhorst plaque found on routine examination associated with significant extracranial carotid disease is shown in Figure 1.4. This women was found to have a severely stenotic and ulcerated lesion in the distal portion of the carotid bulb. At the time of surgery a complex plaque with ulceration and subintimal atheromatous gruel was found.

Figure 1.5 shows a long tight stenosis in the proximal left internal carotid artery of a patient presenting with left hemispheric TIAs and amaurosis fugax of the left eye. At operation (Figure 1.6) a complex plaque with several areas of subintimal hemorrhage and one ulcer located distally were found.

Thrombus overlying a tight stenotic lesion may also be a source of emboli. The patient in Figure 1.7 presented with a series of episodes of

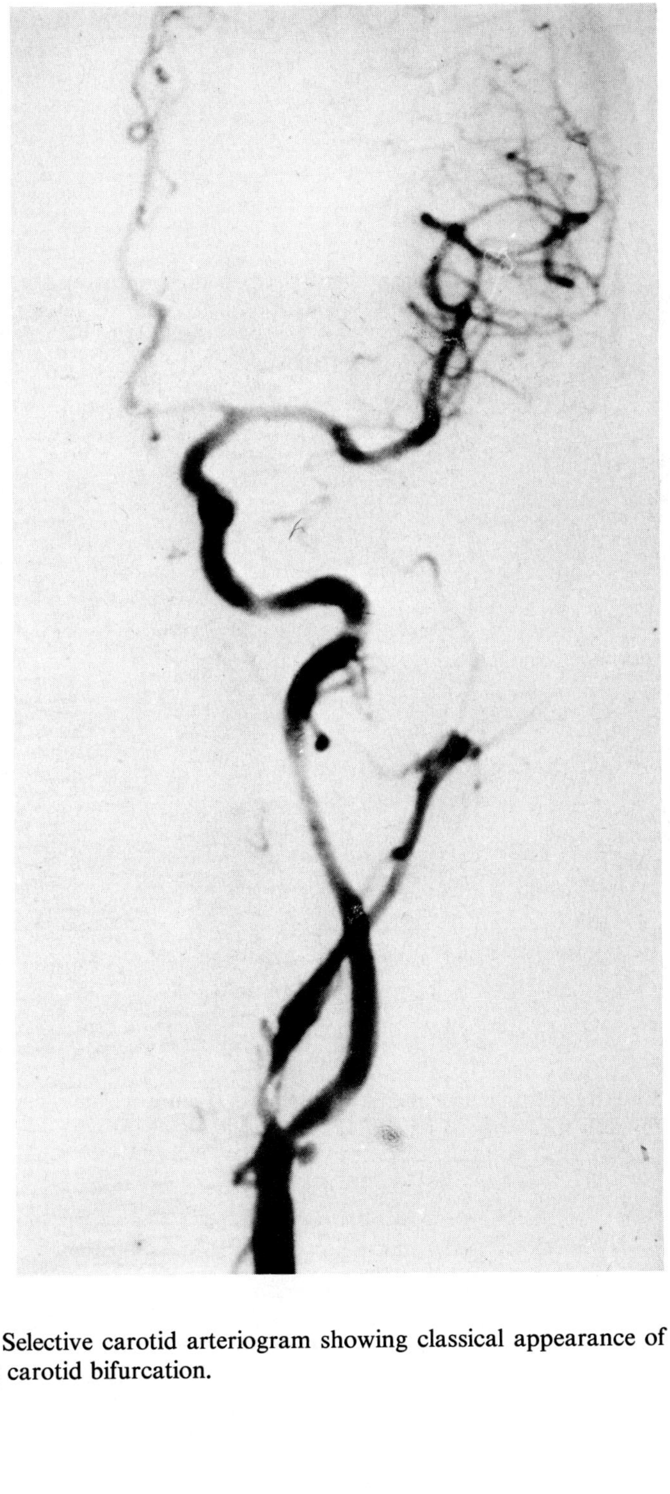

Fig. 1.2. Selective carotid arteriogram showing classical appearance of ulcerated plaque at carotid bifurcation.

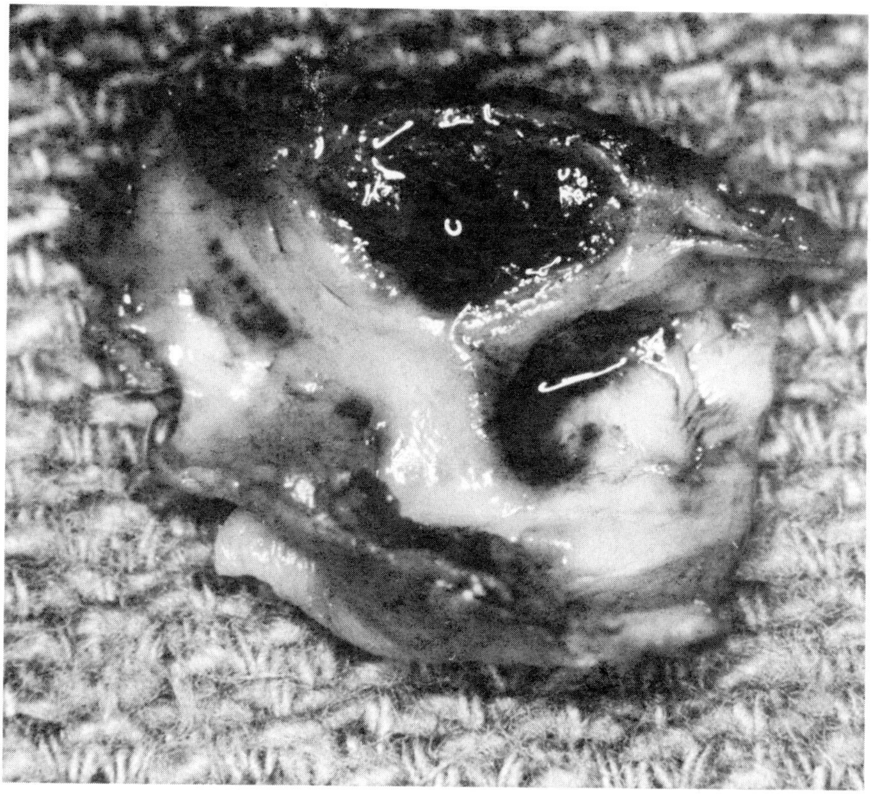

Fig. 1.3. Endarterectomy specimen of patient in Figure 1.2 showing ulcerated plaque with fresh thrombus in base.

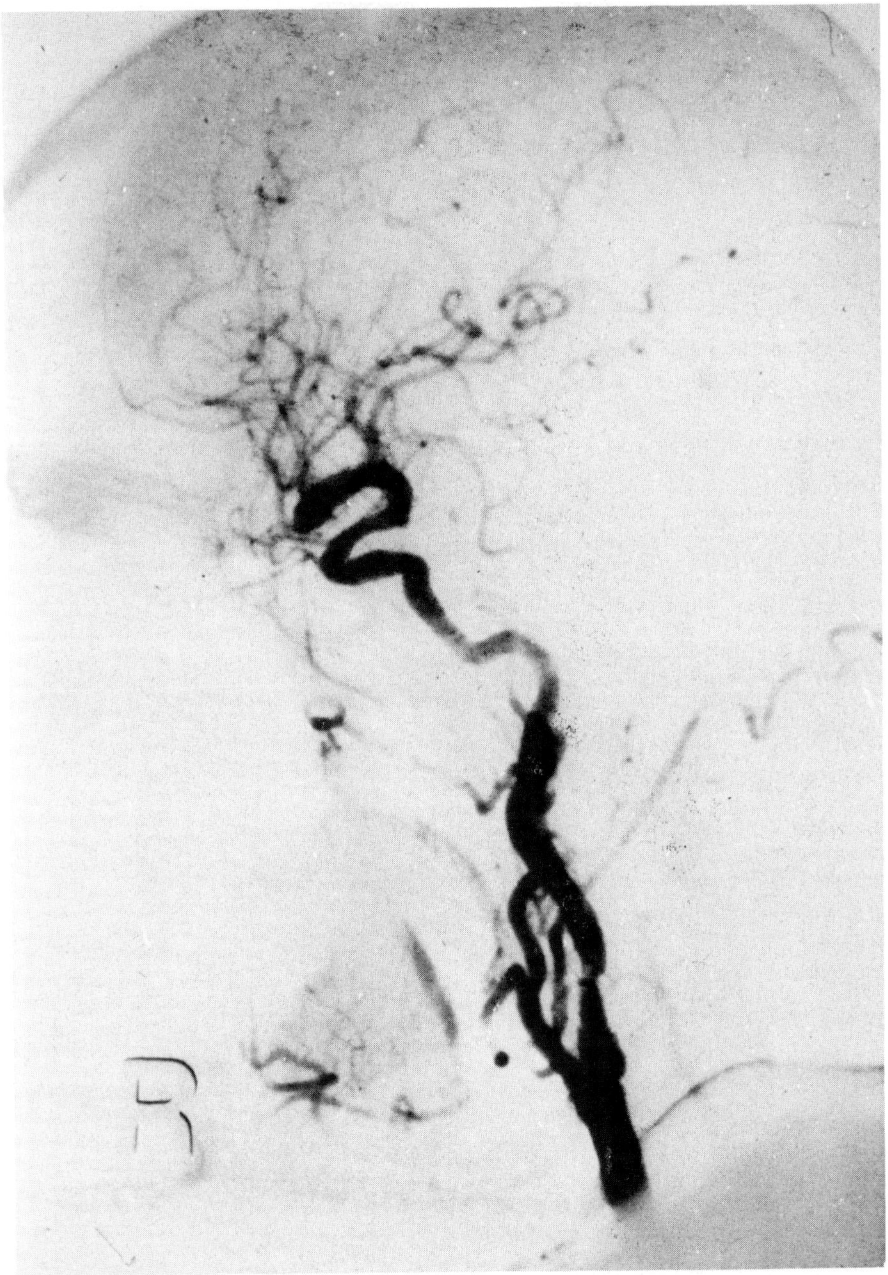

Fig. 1.4. Selective carotid arteriogram showing ulcerated stenotic area in proximal internal carotid artery of patient with asymptomatic Hollenhorst plaque in ipsilateral eye.

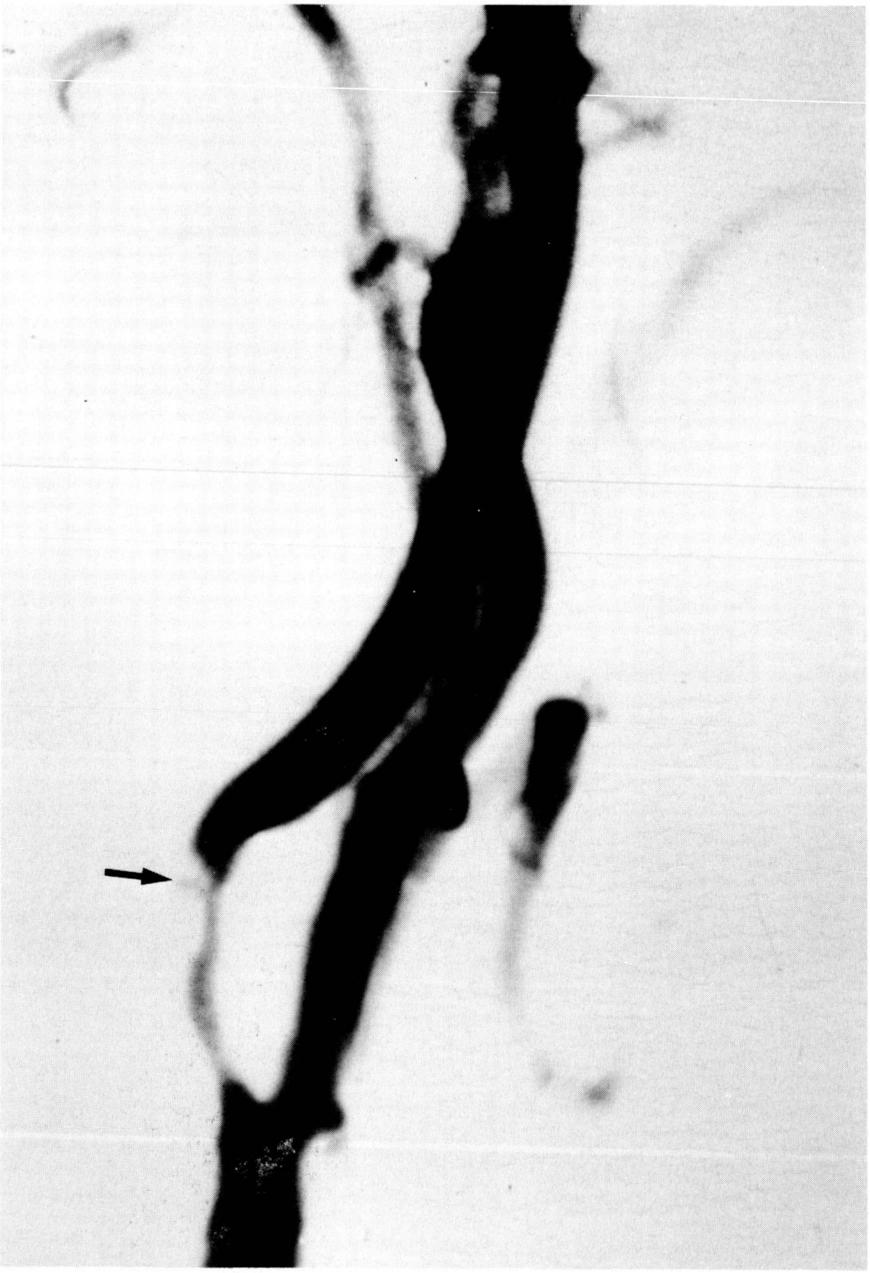

Fig. 1.5. Selective carotid arteriogram in patient with amaurosis fugax left eye and left hemipheric TIAs showing long stenotic area with ulceration (*arrow*) at distal end of plaque.

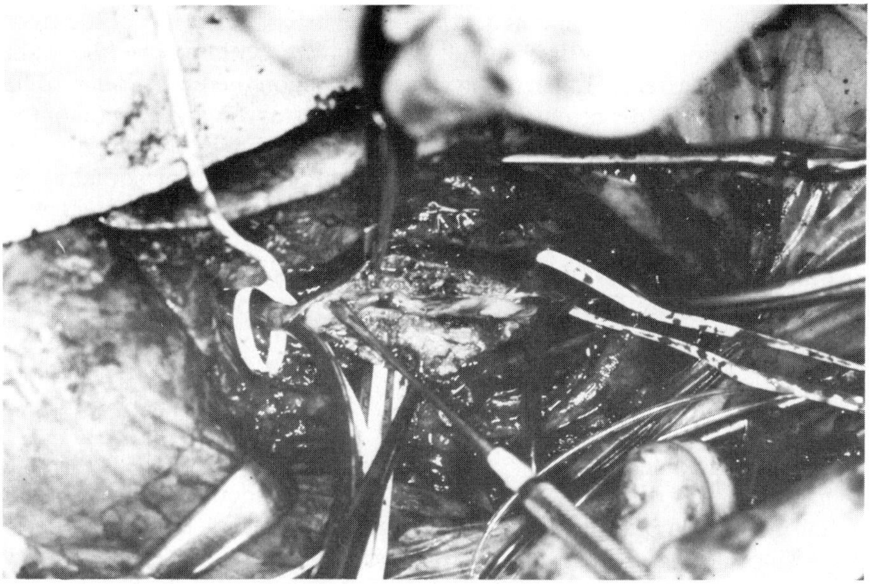

Fig. 1.6. Intraoperative view of patient in Figure 1.5 showing complex plaque with multiple areas of subintimal hemorrhage and ulceration (spatula).

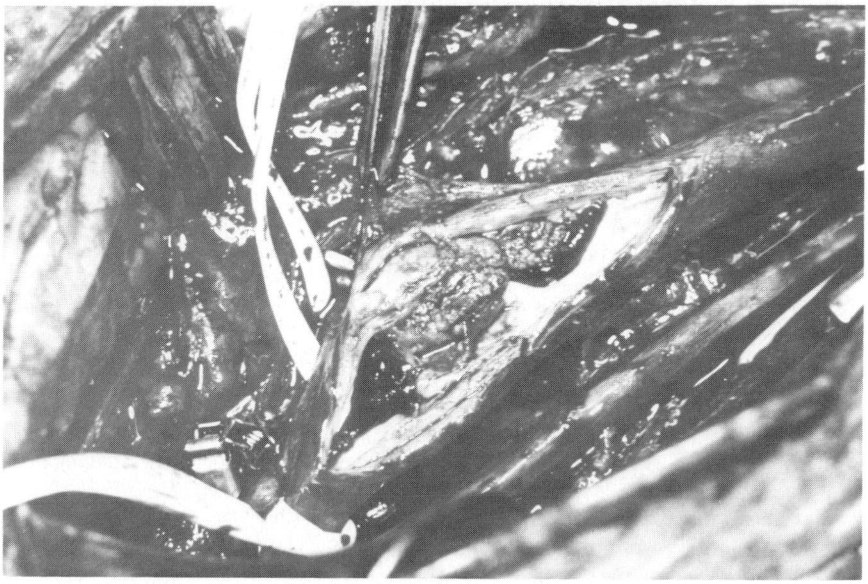

Fig. 1.7. Intraoperative photograph of patient with severe stenosis secondary to complex plaque with overlying thrombus proximal and distal to stenosis. Patient presented with frequent episodes of amaurosis fugax culminating in central retinal artery occlusion of the ipsilateral eye.

amaurosis fugax culminating in central retinal artery occlusion of the right eye. An arteriogram at first suggested complete occlusion of the right internal carotid artery. However, on closer inspection there was found to be evidence of a markedly attenuated lumen in the distal cervical portion of the artery. The patient was explored and was found to have a severe stenosis secondary to a complex plaque with fresh thrombus located proximally and distally to it. Immediately distal to the area of the stenosis the artery was free of disease and thrombus and, in fact, brisk back-bleeding was encountered. Although the patient's vision was not restored by the operative procedure, it prevented a potentially complete and irreversible occlusion of the internal carotid artery.

SUMMARY

In summary there is a large body of clinical evidence suggesting that emboli are an important cause of retinal and cerebral ischemic events. Plaque morphology and surface characteristics can determine the tendency of a plaque to embolize as well as the nature of those emboli. The work of Imparato and Luzby suggests that intraplaque hemorrhage is the most important morphologic characteristic associated with cerebral or ocular syptoms. It is imperative that every physician evaluating patients for ocular ischemia be aware of its relationship with extracranial carotid disease in order to minimize the chance of further visual deterioration or subsequent strokes.

REFERENCES

1. Fisher, C.M.: Observations of the fundus oculi in transient monocular blindness. *Neurology* 9:333, 1959.
2. Hollenhorst, R.W.: Significance of bright plaques in the retinal arterioles. *JAMA* 178:123, 1961.
3. Panum, P.L.: Experimentelle beitrage zurrehre von der embodie. *Arch Pathol Anot* 25:308, 1862.
4. Chiari, H.: Uber das verhalter des teilungsurgswirtels der carotis communis hei der endarteritis chronica deformens. *Ver Otsuh Pathol Ges* 9:326, 1905.
5. Flory, C.M.: Arterial occlusions produced by emboli from carotid aortic atheromatous plaques. *Am J. Pathol* 21:549, 1945.
6. David, N.J., Klintworth, G.K. and Friedberg, S.J.: Fatal atheromatous cerebral embolism associated with bright plaque in the retinal arterioles. *Neurology* 13:708, 1903.
7. Kollarits, C.R., Lubow, M., and Hissong, S.L.: Retinal strokes: I. Incidence of carotid atheromata. *JAMA* 222:1237, 1972.
8. Rosenthal D., Cossman, D. and Seletz, J.: Carotid embolization presenting as total monocular blindness. *Arch Surg* 112:1131, 1977.
9. Winter, W.J.: Atheromatous emboli: A cause of cerebral infarction. *Arch Pathol* 64:137, 1957.

10. Sturgill, B.C. and Netsky, M.G.: Cerebral infarction by atheromatous emboli. *Arch Path* 76:189, 1963.
11. Gunning, A.J., Pickering, G.W., Robb-Smith, A.H.T. and Ross, R.: Mural thrombosis of the carotid artery and subsequent embolism. *OJM* 33:155, 1964.
12. Wood, E.H. and Correll, J.W.: Atheromatous ulceration in major neck vessels as a cause of cerebral embolism. *Acta Radiol* 9:520, 1969.
13. Ehrenfeld, W.K., Hoyt, W.F. and Wylie E.J.: Embolization and transient blindness from carotid atheroma. Surgical considerations, *Arch Surg* 93:787, 1966.
14. Moore, W.S. and Hall A.D.: Importance of emboli from carotid bifurcation in pathogenesis of cerebral ischemic attacks. *Arch Surg* 101:708, 1970.
15. Pessin, M.S., Hinton, R.C., Davis, K.R., Duncan, G.W., Roberson, G.H., Ackerman, R.H. and Mohr, J.P.: Mechanisms of acute carotid stroke. *Ann Neurol* 6:245, 1979.
16. Robbins, S.L., Angell, M. and Kumar W.: *Basic Pathology*. Philadelphia: W.B. Saunders, 1981, pp 260-268.
17. Weismann, R.E.: Plaques and platelets. *Arch Surg* 118:1019, 1983.
18. Jaynes, B.J. and Warren, B.A.: Thrombogenicity of components of atheromatous material. *Arch Pathol Lab Med* 105:353, 1981.
19. Hertzer, N.R., Beven E.G. and Benjamin, S.P.: Ultramicroscopic ulcerations and thrombi of the carotid bifurcation. *Arch Surg* 112:1394, 1977.
20. Imparato, A.M., Riles, T.S., Mintzer, R. and Baumann, F.G.: The importance of hemorrhage in the relationship between gross morphologic characteristics and cerebral symptoms in 376 carotid artery plaques. *Ann Surg* 197:195, 1983.
21. Luzby, R.J., Ferrell, L.D., Ehrenfeld, W.K., Stoney, R.J. and Wiley, E.J.: Carotid plaque hemorrhage: Its role in production of cerebral ischemia. *Arch Surg* 117:1479, 1982.

2

OCULAR ASPECTS OF STA-MCA BYPASS

Robert G. Siekert, M.D.
Thomas P. Kearns, M.D.*
Thoralf Sundt, Jr., M.D.**

The indications for superficial temporal to middle cerebral artery (STA-MCA) bypass include symptoms derived from more than one source: occlusion of the intracranial portion of the internal carotid artery; an inaccessible occlusion of the internal carotid or middle cerebral arteries (commonly stenosis or occlusion of the internal carotid artery in its intracavernous portion); or the result of a preoperative prophylactic procedure performed prior to another operation, for example, for an aneurysm of a major intracranial artery. Of the patients with occlusive lesions, the vast majority, perhaps 80% or more, have operations performed for symptoms caused by occlusion of the intracranial portion of the internal carotid artery. This group commonly experiences ocular symptoms or has ocular involvement.

VISUAL SYMPTOMS

The typical visual symptom is of rather abrupt onset with decreased vision in one or both eyes, frequently diminishing in one portion of the field. This experience has been described as a curtain coming across a portion of the visual field. The vision returns to normal within 15 to 60 minutes. The visual impairment results from decreased blood flow to the retina or to the visual pathways. Although arterial-arterial embolus frequently stems from ulcerated stenosis of the internal carotid artery, in patients with an occluded

*Department of Ophthalmology
and
**Department of Neurosurgery, Mayo Clinic, Rochester, Minnesota

internal carotid artery, the decrease in vision is more likely the consequence of decreased intraocular arterial pressure. Visual loss as a consequence of orthostatic hypotension in the retinal circulation itself, similar to cerebral orthostatism, may clearly be related to a sitting or standing position (1,2). These transient visual symptoms disappear in the majority of patients after STA-MCA bypass.

Some patients comment about a persistent decrease in vision or a film in front of their eye regardless of the position, and their visual acuity may be decreased one or two lines on the chart. One might speculate that the blood flow is decreased just enough to reduce function, but not enough to cause infarction.

A particular kind of visual loss occurring on exposure to bright light with slow return of vision on the involved side has been described (3).

We have seen patients without visual symptoms who have venous stasis retinopathy on examination. Such a finding may alert the examiner to the possibility of carotid occlusive disease.

VENOUS STASIS RETINOPATHY

Venous stasis retinopathy was first described in 1962 by Hedges (4) and in 1963 by Kearns and Hollenhorst (5). This retinopathy consists of punctate areas of capillary dilatation, microaneurysms, small retinal hemorrhages, and dilatation, and darkening and irregularity of the caliber of the major retinal veins (Figs. 2.1, A–C). It resembles diabetic retinopathy and, presumably, therefore, has a similar cause, namely hypoperfusion. In bilateral occlusive disease of the carotid artery, bilateral retinopathy may occur. Venous stasis retinopathy is first seen in the mid-peripheral retina, whereas the early retinal changes of diabetic retinopathy are usually seen in the macula and the posterior pole of the eye. The main difference, however, is that venous stasis retinopathy is unilateral on the side of an occlusive carotid lesion whereas diabetic retinopathy is always bilateral. The presence of low retinal artery pressure is, thus, diagnostic for venous stasis retinopathy, and in most instances will indicate a severely stenotic (over 95%) or occluded internal carotid artery. In patients who have both venous stasis retinopathy and diabetic retinopathy, that is involvement of both eyes with retinopathy, the retinopathy may be worse on the side of the occluded carotid artery.

Occasionally, occlusion of the central retinal vein will be confused with venous stasis retinopathy in that the microaneurysms and punctate dilatation of the capillary arteries may be similar. However, patients with central retinal vein occlusion have more hemorrhage. The veins, while

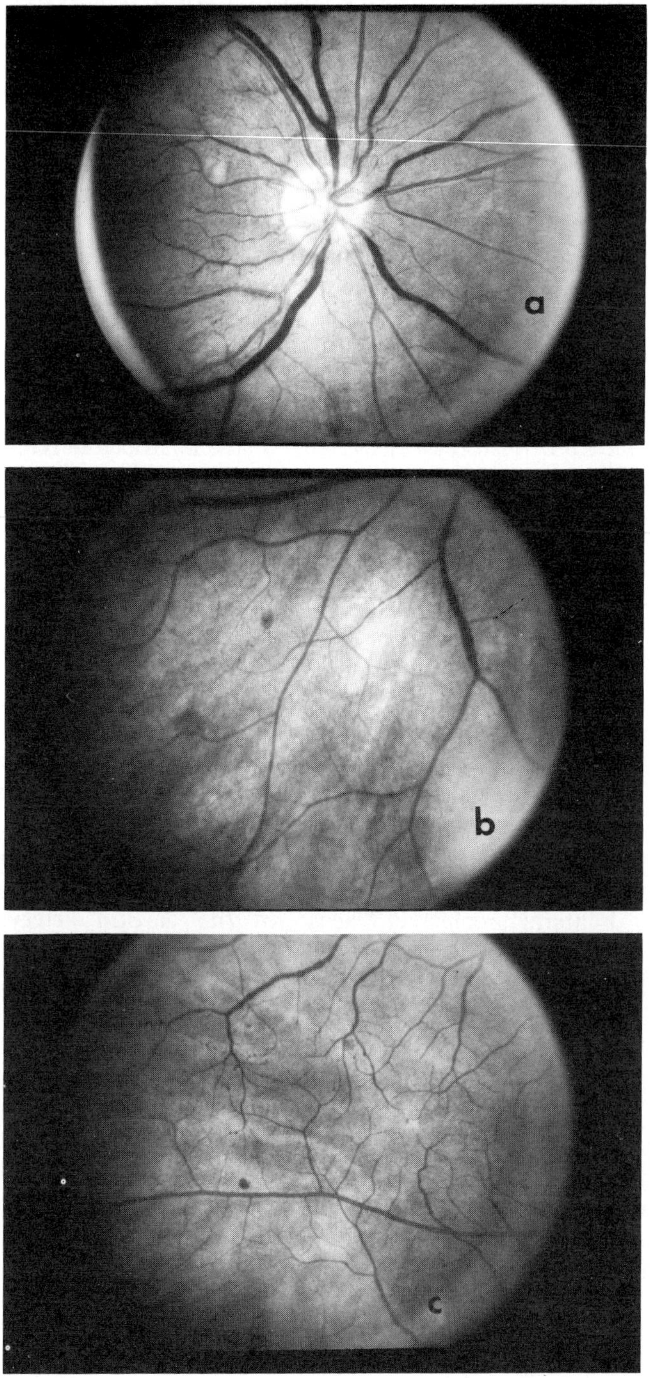

Fig. 2.1. A–C: three views of the same retina prior to operation (Figure continues).

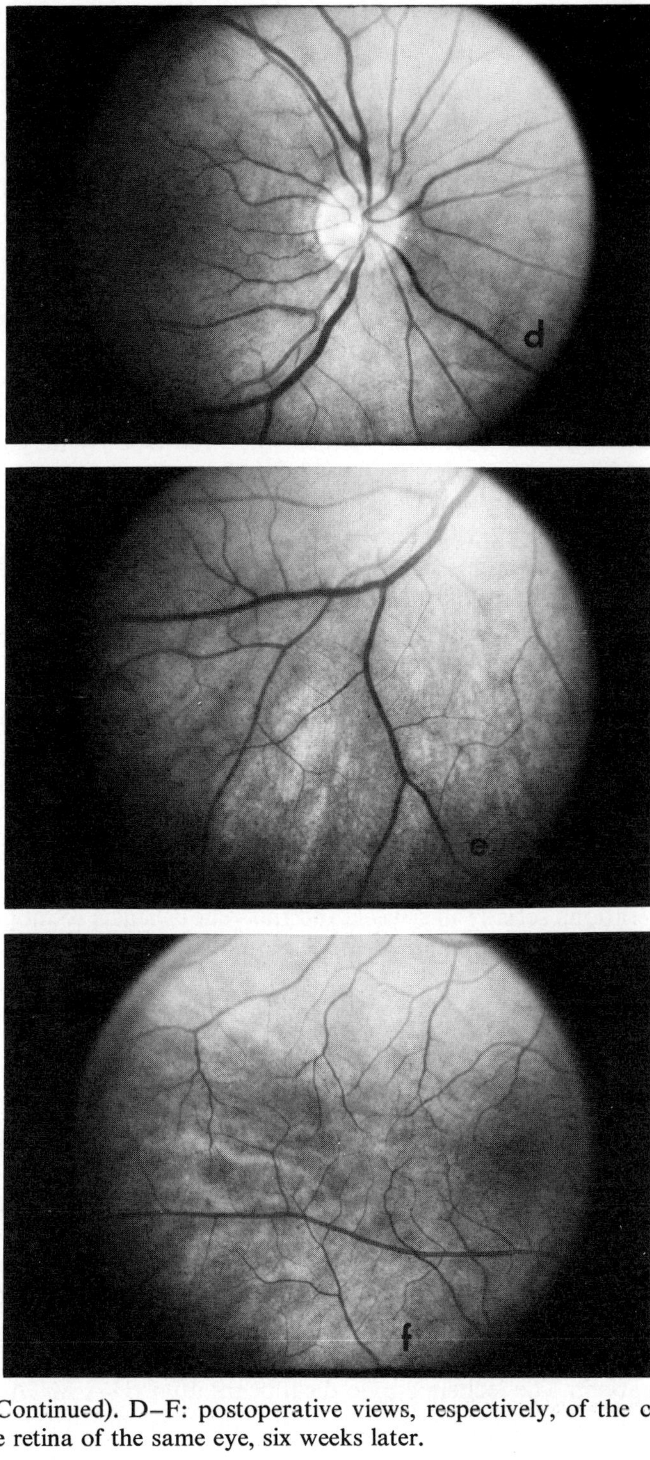

Fig. 2.1 (Continued). D–F: postoperative views, respectively, of the comparable part of the retina of the same eye, six weeks later.

darkened and engorged, do not become irregular in caliber, like sausages, as they do in venous stasis retinopathy. The central retinal artery pressure is normal in retinal vein occlusion.

Soft ischemic exudates may be seen occasionally in patients with occlusion of the carotid artery and these are not specifically part of venous stasis retinopathy but result rather from the occlusion of arterioles.

Patients with venous stasis retinopathy from carotid artery occlusion may continue to have increasing difficulty over time with rubeosis iridis, neovascularization of the anterior chamber angle, secondary glaucoma, and cataract.

The true incidence of venous stasis retinopathy in patients with occlusion of the internal carotid artery is not known, since asymptomatic carotid occlusion often goes undetected. Venous stasis retinopathy may disappear after a bypass operation (6) (Figure 2.1 D–F).

We looked at a group of 72 patients undergoing STA-MCA bypass who had internal carotid occlusion and primarily ocular ischemic symptoms; 25 (35%) had venous stasis retinopathy. Of these 25, 15 had pre- and postoperative examinations; in 10 the venous stasis retinopathy resolved (follow-up examinations from 1 month to 2 years), 3 improved (1 patient was seen 5 days postoperatively), and 2 patients were worse over time. These 2 people suffered from severe neovascularization on the iris with secondary effects. Both had had evidence at time of operation of new vessels; neither had diabetes. In other patients in whom neovascularization was noted but who did not have venous stasis retinopathy, the eye continued to demonstrate increasing ischemic abnormality over time. One patient in the resolution group had bilateral internal carotid artery occlusion and bilateral venous stasis retinopathy. He had his bilateral bypass operations serially in a week and the venous stasis retinopathy had resolved at a four-month postoperative examination.

OCULAR PAIN

Eye pain is occasionally complained of by patients with carotid artery occlusion (1). The pain is within or over the orbit and may spread to the face, and temple; it is worse when the patient is sitting or standing and is reduced or relieved by lying flat. The eye pain is not a common feature occurring perhaps in 5 to 10% of patients with symptoms of carotid occlusion. This pain may be confused with that of secondary glaucoma but the ischemic pain is out of proportion to the slight (if any) elevation of intraocular tension. Of course, glaucoma and ischemic pain may occur in the same patient. The ischemic pain disappears after STA-MCA bypass.

RETINAL ARTERY PRESSURE

Ophthalmodynamometry

Kearns and associates (7) reported on the effect of STA-MCA bypass on the central retinal artery pressures. The compared the relationship of the pressures on the occluded and the non-occluded sides, before and after the operation. The actual mean pressures were converted to percentages, that is, the lower (occluded side) was a percentage of the higher (non-occluded) pressure, using the formula for mean pressure, $S - D/3 + D$ (6). In 22 patients the average pressure on the occluded side was 51% of that of the nonoccluded side prior to operation and 62% after bypass. Several patients showed no change in the pressures with operation, and no attempt was made to correlate any change to the length of time from operation to measurement.

In our current review of 72 patients, with only ocular symptoms, unlike that of Kearns et al., (7) we obtained pre- and postoperative retinal artery measurements in 22. Nineteen had unilateral occlusion of the internal carotid artery and three had bilateral internal carotid occlusion.

After bypass in the 19 patients with unilateral occlusion, 10 had an increase from an average of 32% to an average of 72%; 4 patients showed a decrease in the operative side average (68% to 61%); and 5 patients showed no change in the percentages.

Of the three patients with bilateral occlusion, two had a unilateral operation on the symptomatic side where the pressure was lower, and in both the relative pressure increased significantly (8% to 22%, respectively) on the operated side. In one patient after bilateral operation, the pressures remained equal, with the mean pressures increased 200% from preoperative levels.

Oculoplethysmography

Oculoplethysmography, OPG (Gee), was performed in only two patients before and after bypass. The pressure on the lower (operated) side increased to above the "normal" line after bypass.

DISCUSSION

Halsey and coworkers (8) studied the cerebral blood flow in 19 patients before and after STA-MCA bypass with ^{133}Xe inhalation at rest and during inhalation of CO_2 added to room air. Small differences in blood flow existed between the two sides preoperatively, with the lesser flow on the side of the occluding lesion. They noted that after bypass blood flow increased in both the operated side and the nonoperated side ($p < 0.05$). The increase in cerebral blood flow was greater on the ischemic side after operation. The amount of flow to both hemispheres continued to increase after six months. CO_2 reactivity increased in some patients, more in those with the poorest reactivity prior to operation.

Using the ^{133}Xe inhalation method for cerebral blood flow, Meyer and associates (9) studied 33 patients before and after STA-MCA bypass, 24 with intracranial carotid occlusion or intracranial stenosis, and compared them with two matched, normal, healthy volunteers. Compared to normal controls with values of 76 ± 10 ml/100 g/min of brain flow, preoperative F_1 values in patients were reduced in both the hemispheres. On the side of the occluding carotid lesion, the values were 61.1 ± 11.2 ml/100 g/min ($p > 0.001$). In the contralateral hemispheres, the value was 64.6 ± 10 ml/100 g/min ($p < 0.001$).

The values after STA-MCA bypass were significantly increased. On the bypassed side the mean increase in the hemispheric F_1 value was 12.8% and on the contralateral (nonoperated) side it was 8%. These results indicate that flow to both hemispheres is significantly improved. Most increase was seen in the frontal regions.

Meyer et al. (9) noted that the increases in flow were statistically significant 1–2 weeks after surgery, a trend that continued for 3 months, after which no more change occurred. A tendency for a decrease in flow was noted at 30 months after operation.

Also studied by Meyer and associates were the effects of STA-MCA bypass on cerebral responsiveness to 5% carbon dioxide and to 100% oxygen inhalation. Prior to operation the mean hemispheric vasodilator response to that stimulus was slightly reduced ($+2.5 \pm 2.9\ \Delta\%\ F_1/\Delta$mm Hg $PECO_2$) compared to values for age-matched normal controls (+3.5 ± 1.7%). This impairment in reactivity was not significantly improved after bypass. Compared to normal volunteers, vasoconstrictive responses to 100% oxygen inhalation were slightly impaired prior to bypass and were not significantly altered after surgery.

Baron et al. report the reversal of hemodynamic cerebral ischemia studied by ^{15}O positron emission tomography (10), after a bypass procedure. They comment that tissue with poor blood supply may not function but still remains viable.

It is apparent from our observations that successful STA-MCA bypass resulting in patent vessels is associated with an improved ocular status. Included are the observed changes in venous stasis retinopathy and increased central retinal artery pressures as well as the disappearance of the ocular pain and obscuration of vision. The last mentioned is certainly the most important to the patient.

REFERENCES

1. Sundt, T.M., Siekert, R.G., Piepgras, D.G., Sharbrough, F.W., and Houser, O.W.: Bypass surgery for vascular disease of the carotid system. *Mayo Clin. Proc.* 51:677, 1976.
2. Russell, R.W.R., and Page, N.G.R.: Critical perfusion of brain and retina. *Brain* 106:419, 1983.
3. Furlan, A.J., Whisnant, J.P., and Kearns, T.P.: Unilateral visual loss in bright light - An unusual symptom of carotid artery occlusive disease. *Arch. Neurol.* 36:675, 1979.
4. Hedges, T.R., Jr.: Ophthalmoscopic findings in internal carotid artery occlusion. *Johns Hopkins Med. J.* 111:89, 1962.
5. Kearns, T.P., Hollenhorst, R.W.: Venous-stasis retinopathy of occlusive disease of the carotid artery. *Proc. Staff Meet. Mayo Clin.* 38:304, 1963.
6. Kearns, T.P., Younge, B.P., and Piepgras, D.G.: Resolution of venous stasis retinopathy after carotid artery bypass surgery. *Mayo Clin. Proc.* 55:342, 1980.
7. Kearns, T.P., Siekert, R.G., and Sundt, T.M., Jr.: The ocular aspects of bypass surgery of the carotid artery. *Mayo Clin. Proc.* 54:3, 1979.
8. Halsey, J.H., Jr., Morawetz, R.B., and Blauenstein, V.W.: The hemodynamic effect of STA-MCA bypass. *Stroke* 13:163, 1982.
9. Meyer, J.S., Nokajima, S., et al.: Redistribution of cerebral blood flow following STA-MCA bypass in patients with hemispheric ischemia. *Stroke* 13:774, 1982.
10. Baron, J.C., Bousser, M.G., Rey, A., Guillard, A., Comar, D., and Castaigne, P.: Reversal of focal "misery-perfusion syndrome" by extra-intracranial arterial bypass in hemodynamic cerebral ischemia, a case study with ^{15}O positron emission tomography. *Stroke* 12:454, 1981.

3

EYE PATHOLOGY SECONDARY TO NONATHEROSCLEROTIC DISEASE OF THE CAROTID ARTERY

E. Kieffer, M.D.*
C. Ruotolo, M.D.*
Y. Bensaïd, M.D.*
G. Rancurel, M.D.**

Atherosclerotic lesions of the carotid bifurcation probably represent the bulk of everyday practice in many vascular centers. However the clinical significance of nonatherosclerotic disease of the carotid artery should not be underestimated, since hemispheric and ocular manifestations may be just as threatening as those from atherosclerotic lesions. From 1979 to 1983 we performed a total of 1099 carotid reconstructions (Table 3.1). Nonatherosclerotic disease of the carotid artery was treated surgically in a total of 183 cases (16.6%). Most of these instances were isolated nonatherosclerotic lesions while 52 were combined atherosclerotic and nonatherosclerotic lesions.

The purpose of this chapter is to describe the main pathological and clinical features of nonatherosclerotic diseases of the carotid artery and to emphasize the surgical indications and special techniques of their operative management.

ARTERIAL LESIONS

A variety of nonatherosclerotic lesions of the carotid artery may be encountered. Their types and usual location are listed in Table 3.2.

From the *Vascular Surgery Service and **Department of Neurology, Groupe Hospitalier Pitié-Salpétrière, Paris, France.

TABLE 3.1. Carotid artery reconstruction (1979–1983)

Condition	*N*	%
Atherosclerotic disease	916	83.4
Nonatherosclerotic disease	131	11.9
Combined	52	4.7
Total	1099	100

TABLE 3.2. Types and usual location of nonatherosclerotic disease of carotid artery

Topography	*Common Pathology*
Common carotid artery	Radiation arteritis
	Takayasu's arteritis
Carotid bifurcation	Embolism
Internal carotid artery	Kinking
	Fibromuscular dysplasia
	Dissection
	Aneurysm

Kinking

Excessive length of the internal carotid artery resulting in tortuosity (Figures 3.1 and 3.2) or coiling (Figures 3.1B and 3.3) is frequently found in angiograms performed for nonvascular indications, even in children and young adults. These abnormalities are considered to be congenital in origin and probably have no clinical significance. Obstruction of the internal carotid artery secondary to acute angulation (kinking) (Figures 3.1C, D and 3.4) is usually considered result of aging, atherosclerotic changes in the aortic arch and its branches, and possibly systemic hypertension. A few authors (1) deny any clinical significance to these lesions because they are also found in normal, asymptomatic, individuals. In addition their cause-effect relationship in symptomatic patients is often difficult to prove. However most workers now recognize that isolated kinking of the internal carotid artery may be responsible for hemispheric or ocular symptoms in a significant number of cases (2, 3, 4). Carotid kinks have been the most common nonatherosclerotic carotid lesion in our surgical experience.

Such lesions may indeed have hemodynamic consequences, especially in the presence of bilateral or associated lesions, including kinking of the proximal vertebral artery. Clinical consequences usually include symptoms of carotid or vertebrobasilar insufficiency. A positional factor is often

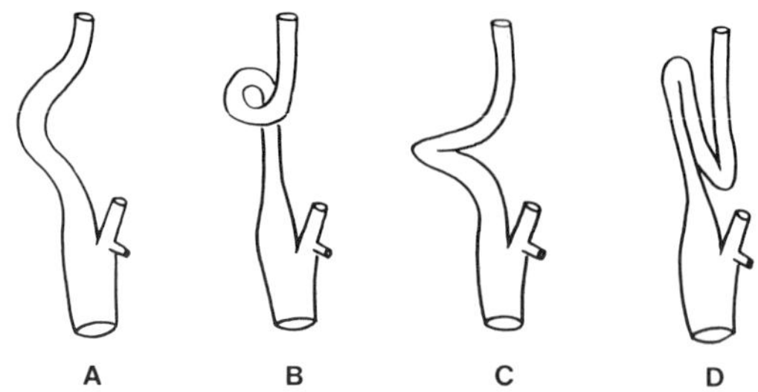

Fig. 3.1. Schematic drawing of tortuosity (**A**), coiling (**B**) and kinking (**C** and **D**) of the internal carotid artery.

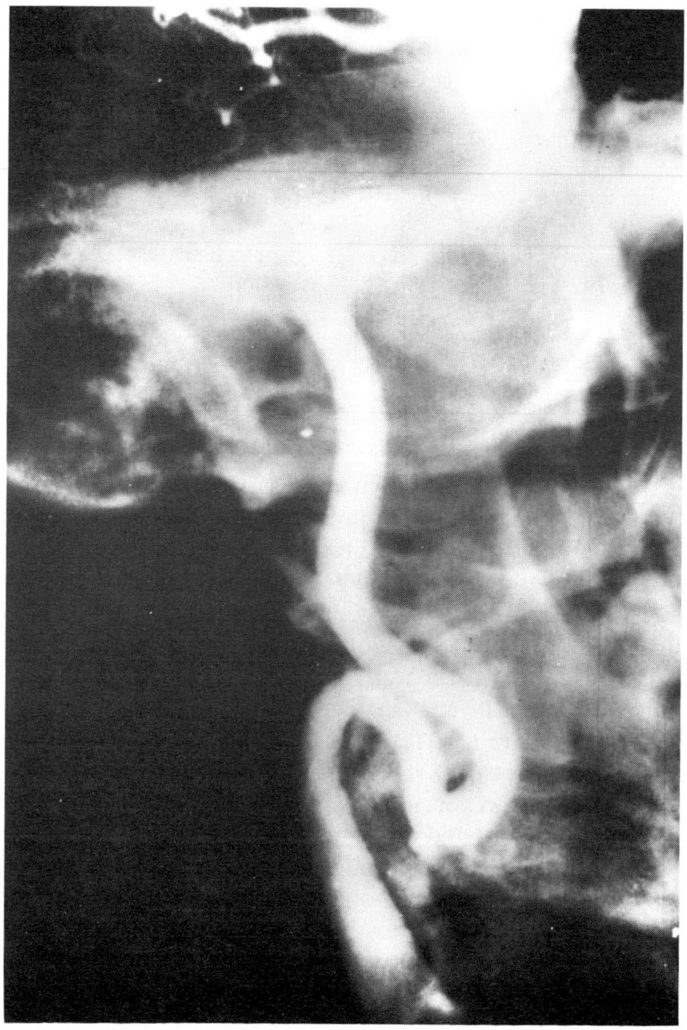

Fig. 3.2. Arteriogram showing marked tortuosity of the internal carotid artery.

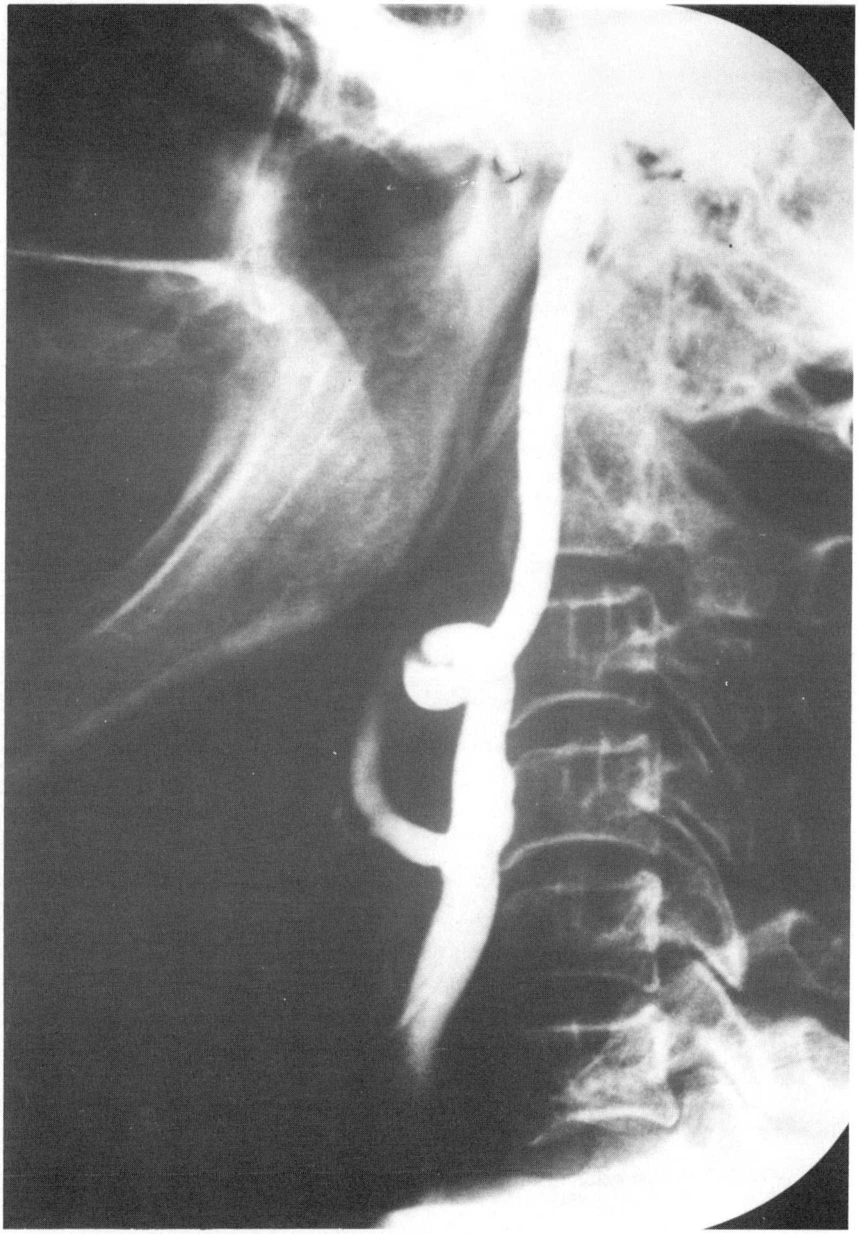

Fig. 3.3. Arteriogram showing coiling of the internal carotid artery.

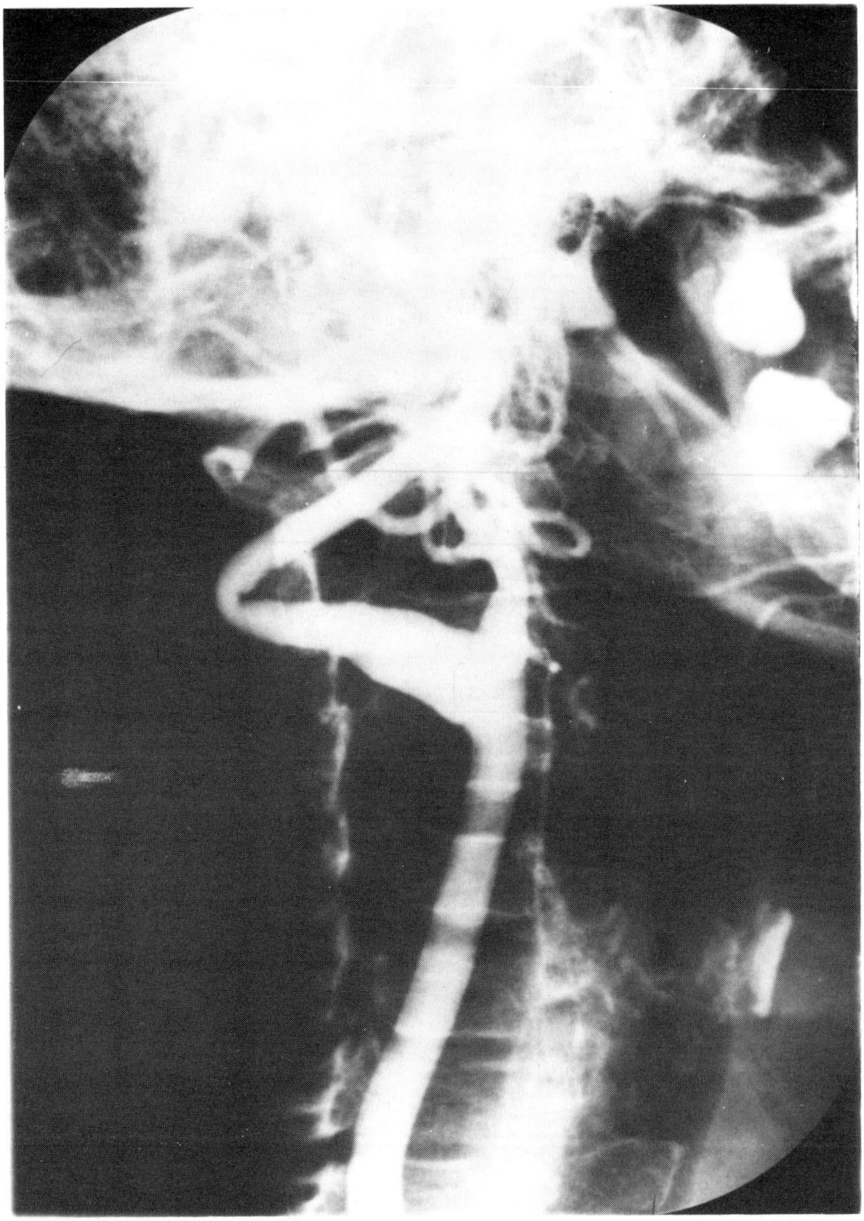

Fig. 3.4. Arteriogram showing kinking of the internal carotid artery.

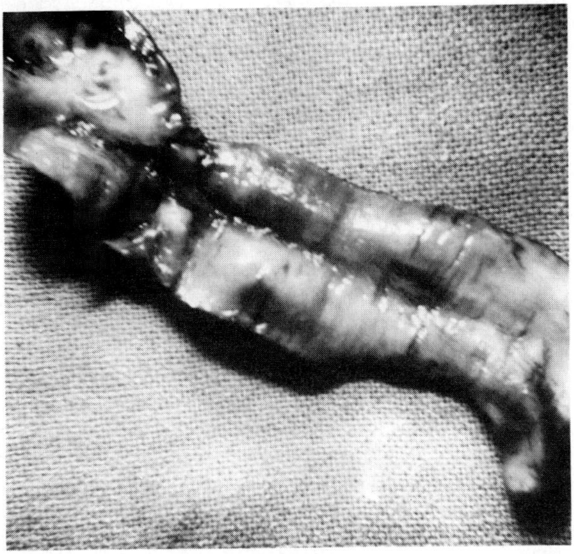

Fig. 3.5. Resected specimen showing marked intimal alterations at point of kinking.

present in these cases and may be proved by angiograms or noninvasive testing. These may demonstrate acute stenosis or even complete occlusion of the internal carotid artery produced by extreme positioning of the head and neck.

Furthermore, hemodynamic strains may result in disease of the arterial wall, which in turn may cause thromboembolic complications leading to hemispheric or ocular symptoms. All of the following have been found in our patients by direct examination of the resected specimen: (1) intimal lesions, with and without ulceration and/or mural thrombosis (Figures 3.4, 3.5); (2) aneurysms, occurring either as a poststenotic dilatation leading to a fusiform aneurysm or as a jet-lesion leading to a sacciform aneurysm; and (3) dissections, usually beginning at the distal part of the kink, characterized by intimal lesions related to the peculiar fragility of the arterial wall and turbulent flow inside the artery. These findings suggest that kinking of the internal carotid artery should not be considered a benign and incidental lesion.

Fibromuscular Dysplasia

Although genetic, mechanical and hormonal factors have been incriminated, fibromuscular dysplasia is probably congenital in origin, with a large predominance of young or middle-aged female patients (5, 6). Both

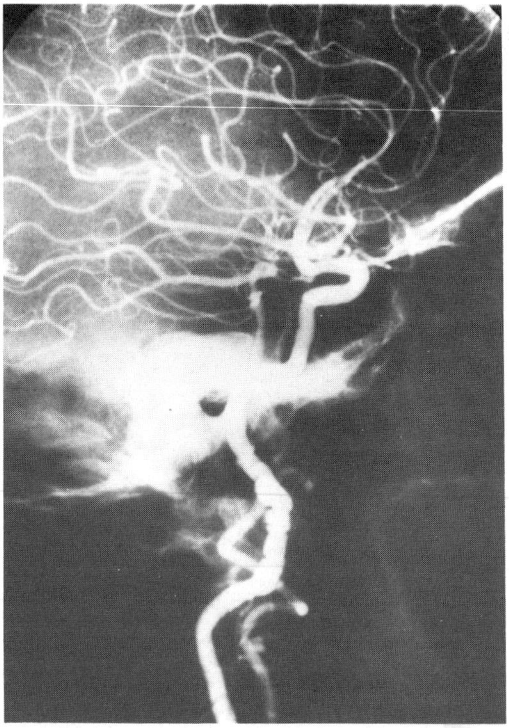

Fig. 3.6. Arteriogram showing the typical "string of beads" appearance in fibromuscular dysplasia of the internal carotid artery.

internal carotid arteries are usually involved, with vertebral artery lesions and even intracranial berry aneurysms associated in a substantial number of cases. Involvement of the extracranial arteries by fibromuscular dysplasia is second in frequency to lesions of the renal arteries, which have been recognized much earlier and whose clinical consequences are certainly more significant due to renovascular hypertension.

The angiographic pattern of the disease is highly characteristic, with the classical "string of beads" appearance affecting the middle and sometimes distal part of the extracranial internal carotid artery (Figure 3.6). In a few cases a less characteristic appearance with long or short tubular stenosis may be present (Figure 3.7). This may cause difficulties in proper diagnosis unless lesions in the contralateral carotid artery or other locales have a more typical appearance. Localized fusiform or sacciform macroaneurysms may also be encountered.

Although an unknown but probably large number of fibrodysplastic lesions of the carotid artery remain completely asymptomatic, it is commonly recognized that clinical symptoms may be caused by fibromuscular dysplasia, either on a hemodynamic or on a thromboembolic basis. Hypoperfusion may be secondary to stenotic intraluminal rings or

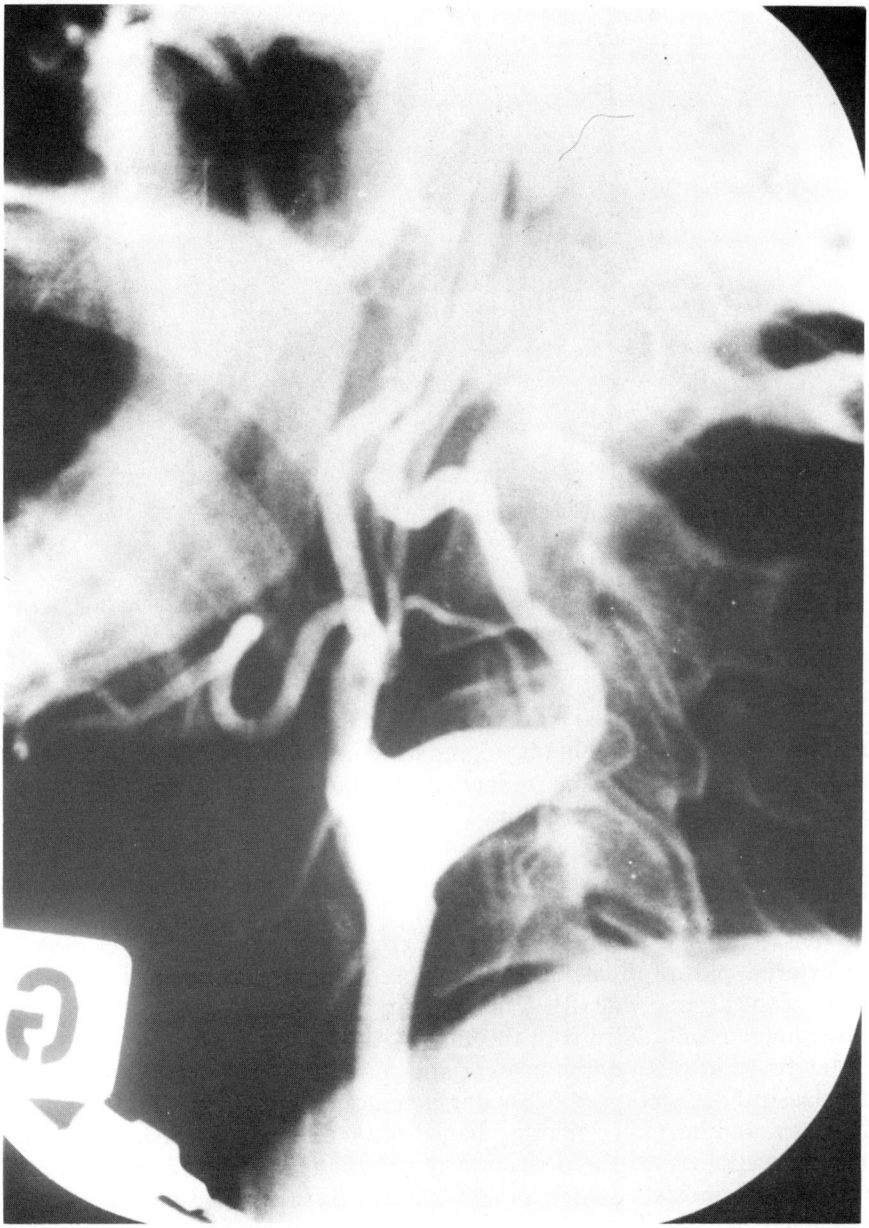

Fig. 3.7. Angiogram showing spontaneous dissection of the internal carotid artery originating at the tip of the carotid bulb.

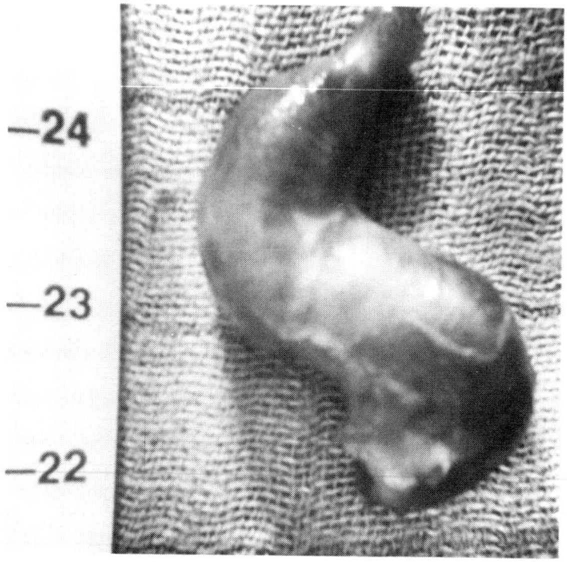

Fig. 3.8. Resected specimen in the same patient showing fusiform dilatation of the artery due to the dissecting hematoma.

the frequently associated kinking of the internal carotid artery. Platelet aggregates or even thrombi may complicate intimal lesions, with or without micro or macroaneurysms. Finally, spontaneous dissection may also complicate fibrodysplastic lesions (7).

Spontaneous Dissection

Dissections of the internal carotid artery are caused by a cleavage in the external part of the media due to loosening of the muscular and elastic fibers of the arterial wall (8). A double lumen is thus created, with the outer false lumen usually filled with thrombus. An intimal tear such as is seen in aortic dissections is seldom present and most cases closely correspond to the classical description of dissecting hematomas. Although fibromuscular dysplasia and hormonal therapy have been incriminated in selected cases, the exact etiology of the dissection remains unknown in the majority of cases. Cystic medial necrosis as seen in aortic dissection has been present in only a few patients. In our patients, dissection often initiated from the distal part of a carotid kink, either at the tip of the carotid bulb (Figures 3.7, 3.8) or before the entrance of the artery in the skull. This suggests the importance of mechanical factors in determining the starting point of a dissection.

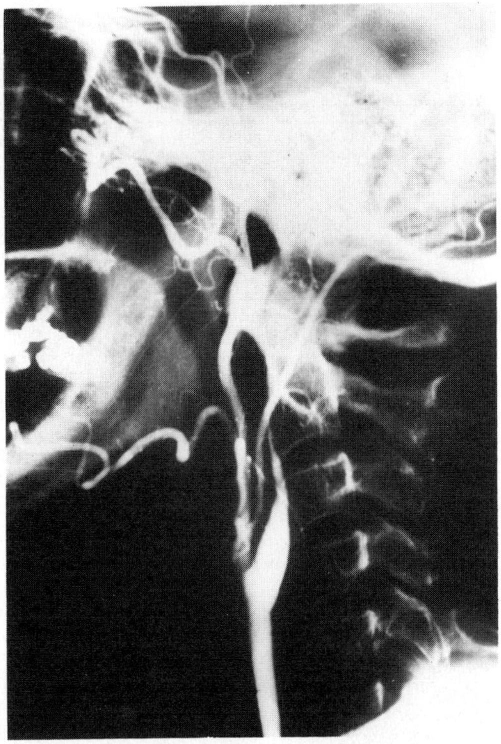

Fig. 3.9. Arteriogram showing typical string-like appearance in an acute dissection of the internal carotid artery.

The clinical consequences and angiographic appearance of dissections are easily explained by the nature of the lesion and its several possible anatomical evolutions. In a few cases with a large entry and exit tear and a patent false lumen, the angiographic appearance is very similar to that of an aortic dissection with slight dilatation of the artery and the presence of a longitudinal intimal flap inside the artery. However the usual early angiographic appearance is that of a typical dissecting hematoma, with a long, tapered, string-like reduction in the caliber of the inner lumen extending from the tip of the carotid bulb up to the site of entrance of the internal carotid artery into the skull (Figure 3.9). In a few cases this lesion may progress rapidly to complete occlusion (Figure 3.10). In the majority of cases however, serial angiograms show spontaneous resolution in a few weeks or months, with return to a near-normal appearance of the carotid lumen. This possibility along with the usual technical difficulties of direct repair, has been the basis for conservative treatment of acute carotid dissections. However a few cases may ultimately progress to late dilatation of the artery, leading to localized sacciform aneurysms, with their attendant

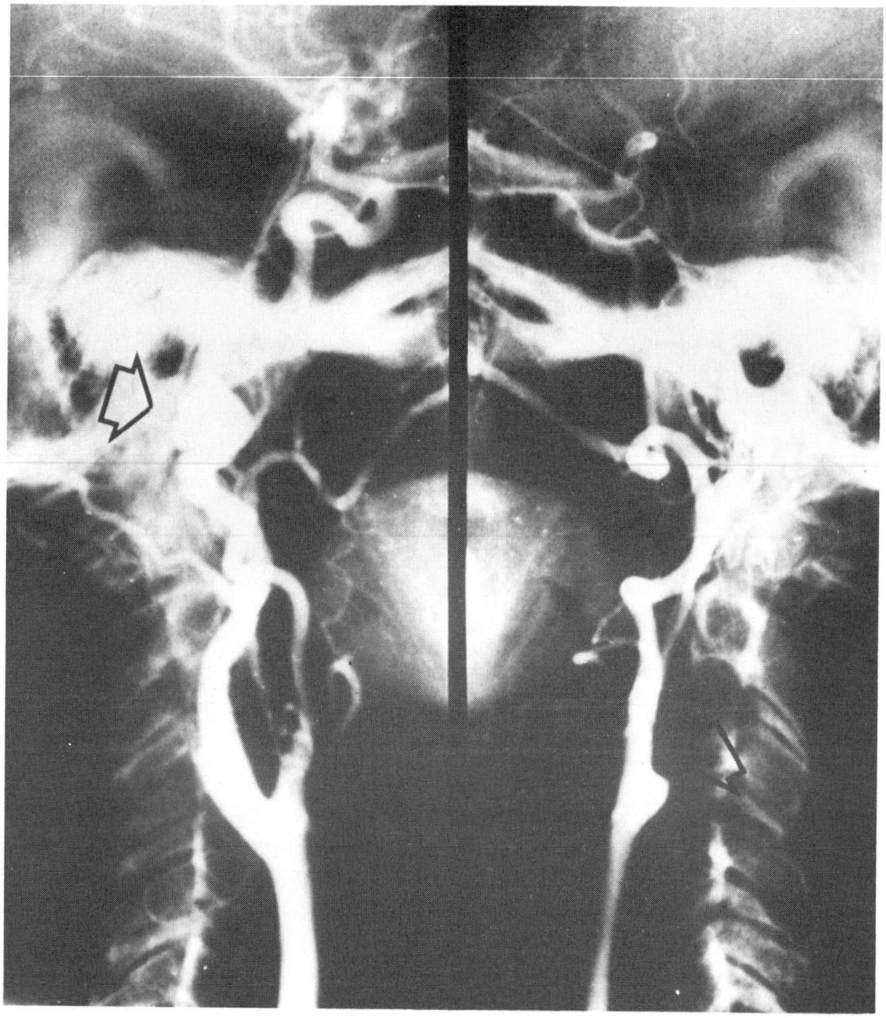

Fig. 3.10. Follow-up arteriogram showing the evolution of a patient with bilateral dissection of internal carotid artery. Pictured at left a sacciform aneurysm has developed. The other side has progressed to a complete occlusion.

risk of thromboembolic complications (Figure 3.10). This justifies the need for a long-term angiographic follow-up of these patients.

Aneurysms

Although infrequent, aneurysms of the carotid artery may have a diverse etiology (9-12). Spontaneous aneurysms of the internal carotid

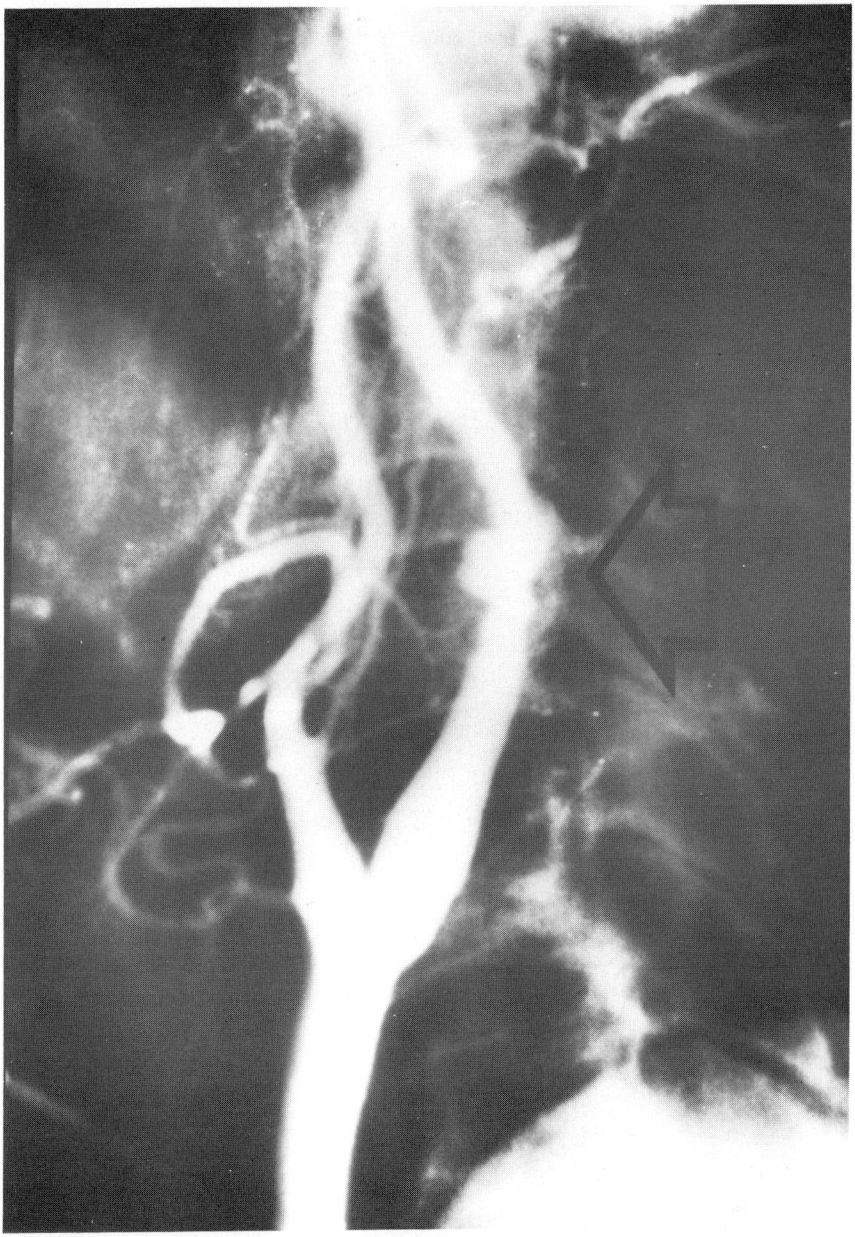

Fig. 3.11. Arteriogram showing a small localized aneurysm of the internal carotid artery in a patient with fibromuscular dysplasia.

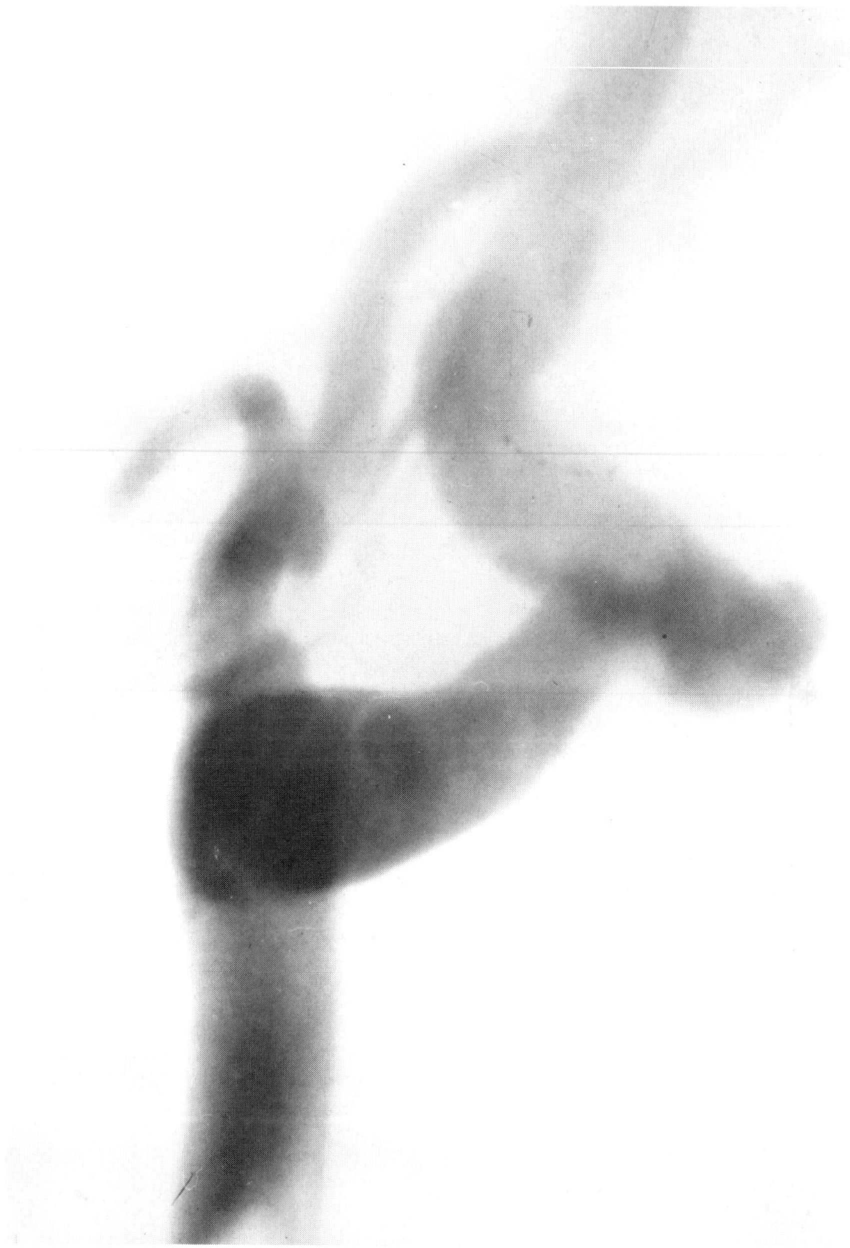

Fig. 3.12. Follow-up arteriogram showing localized dilatation distal to a kink in a patient with spontaneous dissection of the internal carotid artery.

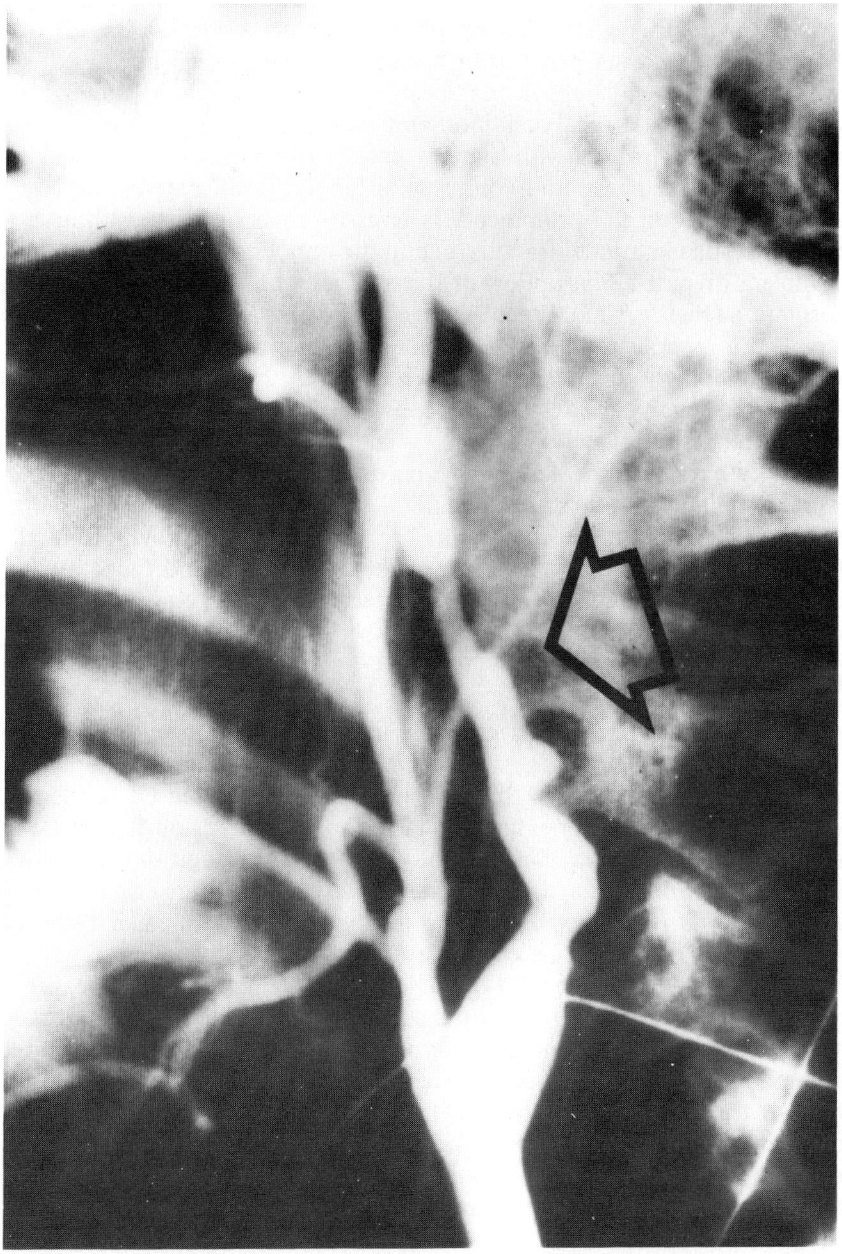

Fig. 3.13. Arteriogram showing aneurysm of the internal carotid artery secondary to nonpenetrating trauma.

artery, either sacciform or fusiform, may be secondary to fibromuscular dysplasia (Figure 3.11), infection, or spontaneous dissection (Figure 3.12). Aneurysms following penetrating trauma are rarely seen nowadays since such a condition usually leads to surgical exploration or angiography, depending on the clinical condition and localization of the injury. However nonpenetrating trauma with hyperextension and rotation of the neck may cause acute stretching and compression of the distal part of the internal carotid artery on the prominent transverse process of C1. Although this usually results in intimal fracture(s) and thrombotic occlusion of the artery, complete or partial disruption of the arterial wall may lead to aneurysm formation (Figure 3.13). Postoperative aneurysms also constitute a rare but significant complication of carotid endarterectomy, especially when patch graft angioplasty has been used. Infection may be present in early cases, whereas mechanical factors are considered to be responsible for late aneurysmal formation.

Whatever their etiology and anatomical appearance, carotid aneurysms usually result in thromboembolic complications, leading to hemispheric or ocular manifestations as the usual presenting symptoms. Less frequently, large or infected aneurysms may rupture and those involving the distal part of the internal carotid artery may cause compression of the neighboring cranial nerves.

Radiation Arteritis

Radiation arteritis is seen with increasing frequency in long-term survivors of neck cancer, who have had radio therapy alone or in combination with surgery. Such patients have an increased incidence of stroke and carotid artery disease (13). The arterial lesion is fibrotic and sometimes calcified in nature and may be histologically difficult to distinguish from standard atherosclerotic lesions. In some cases it may be associated with involvement of the neighboring structures, namely skin, subcutaneous tissues, muscles, and even upper airway leading to technical difficulties in the management of some patients (Figure 3.14). Localization of the arterial damage depends on the topography of the radiation field, any segment of the common or internal carotid artery being potentially vulnerable (Figures 3.15, 3.16). Stenotic lesions of varying degrees may lead to thromboembolic complications and progress to occlusion, often involving both common or internal carotid arteries. In such cases extreme hypoperfusion may be the cause of severe ocular manifestations similar to those described in Takayasu's arteritis.

Takayasu's Arteritis

At the beginning of this century Takayasu, a Japanese ophthalmologist, described a retinal vascular disease of unknown origin in a young

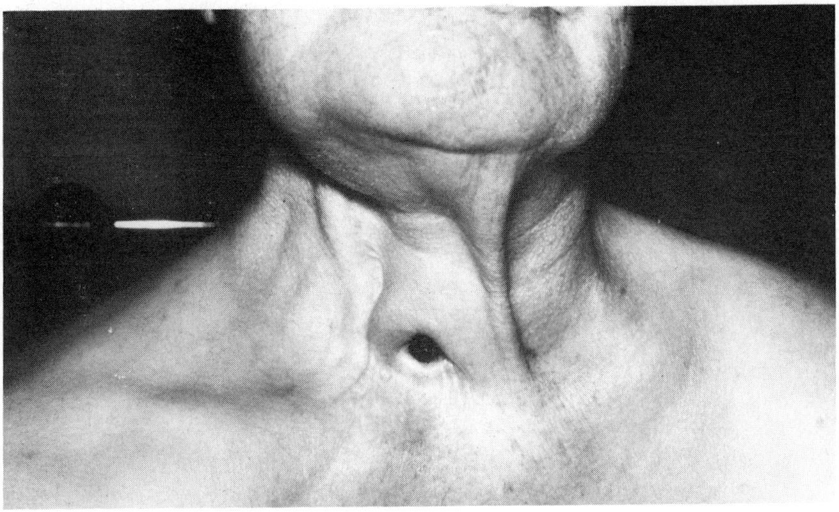

Fig. 3.14. Appearance of the neck of a patient 12 years after combined resection and radiotherapy of a laryngeal cancer. Both common carotid arteries are occluded and there is extensive neck induration in addition to a permanent tracheostomy.

woman. He did not recognize the involvement of the great vessels in his patient, and it was Onishi who established a correlation between vascular occlusive disease and the ocular manifestations in the discussion following Takayasu's presentation. For several decades, Takayasu's arteritis was considered as a rare disease, affecting young female patients coming from the Far East exclusively. Involvement of the proximal intrathoracic great vessels and the presence of a biological inflammatory syndrome were deemed essential to diagnosis. Since that time, although its etiology has remained unknown, the disease has been recognized with increasing frequency throughout the world, including male patients also. Involvement of the entire aorta and its visceral branches is frequent and highly significant in terms of prognosis. Furthermore it has been realized that patients may first be seen in the chronic postinflammatory phase, with arterial lesions representing the chronic sequelae of the acute arteritis (14).

Although a strong intimal fibrotic reaction is usually present, arterial lesions begin and predominate in the adventitia and external part of the media (Figure 3.17). Lymphocyte infiltrates and giant cells may be present in acute lesions. These lesions affect mainly the common carotid arteries (Figure 3.18) and may progress uneventfully to segmental or extensive occlusion of these vessels. In the most advanced cases cerebral and ocular manifestations are secondary to severe hypoperfusion and may be

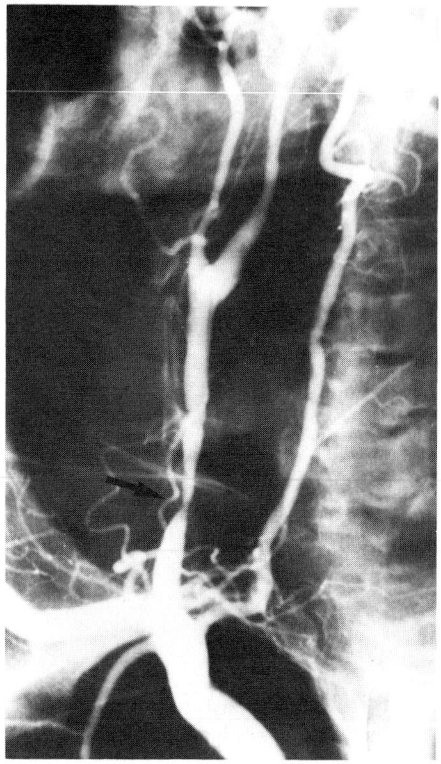

Fig. 3.15. Arteriogram showing stenosis of the common carotid artery in a patient who underwent low cervical irradiation for metastatic lymph nodes.

associated with other manifestations of facial ischemia, including jaw claudication, facial atrophy and even ulceration of the palate, nose or ear (15).

Embolism

Emboli of cardiac origin, whatever their cause and nature may be, usually progress to distal cerebral or ocular vessels. Rarely a large embolus may stop in the carotid bifurcation. We have seen a few such cases causing typical optico-pyramidal syndrome.

OCULAR MANIFESTATIONS

The frequency and nature of ocular manifestations of isolated nonatherosclerotic disease of the carotid artery are shown in table 3.3 and 3.4. In the whole series of 131 patients, 30 had ocular symptoms, for an

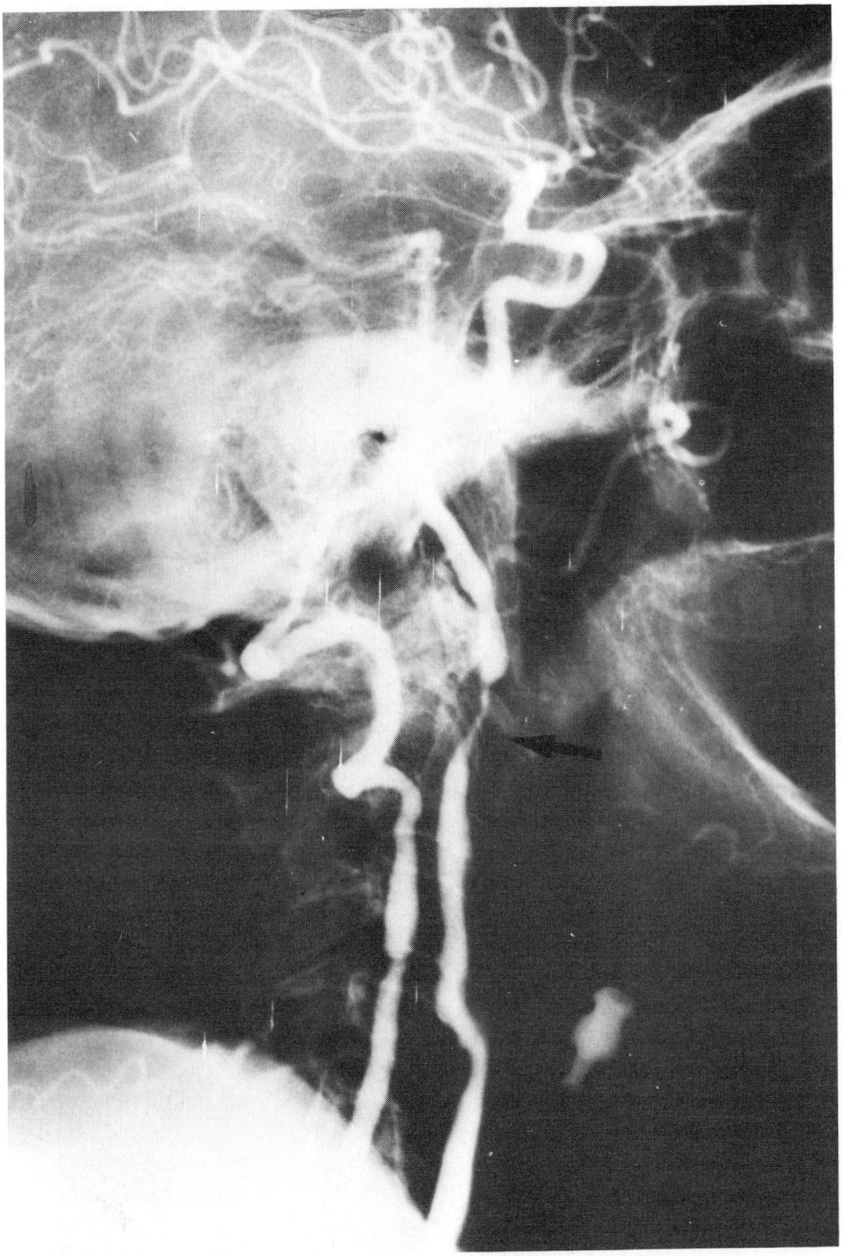

Fig. 3.16. Angiogram showing tight stenosis of the distal internal carotid artery in a patient irradiated for tonsilar carcinoma.

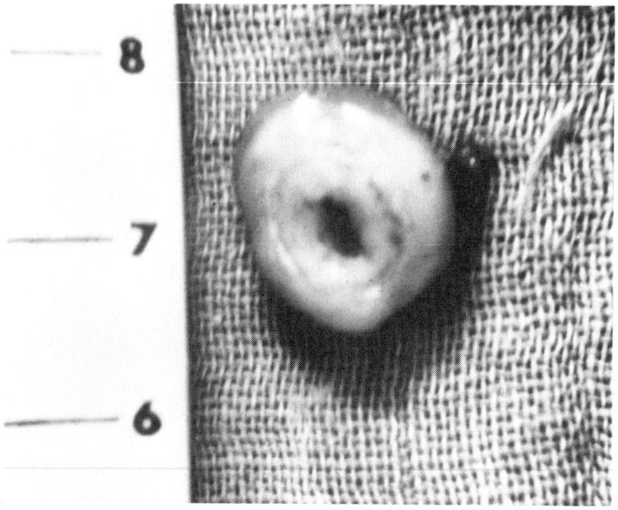

Fig. 3.17. Cross-sectional gross appearance of a resected carotid in a patient with Takayasu's arteritis.

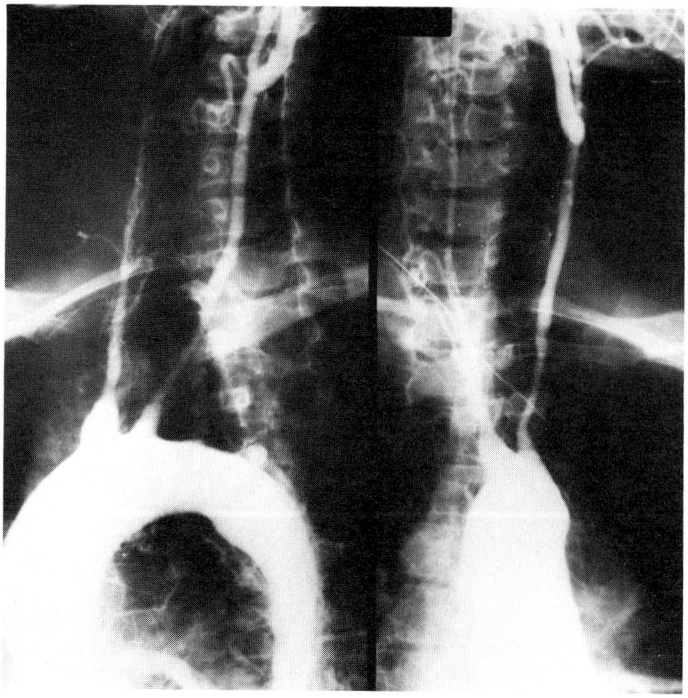

Fig. 3.18. Arteriogram showing extensive involvement of the intrathoracic great vessels in a patient with Takayasu's arteritis.

TABLE 3.3. Incidence of symptoms in isolated, nonatherosclerotic, carotid disease

Disease	*N*	*Ocular manifestations*	%	*Associated cerebral symptoms*	%
Kinking	43	4	9.3	2	50.0
Fibromuscular dysplasia	23	8	34.8	2	25.0
Dissection	17	3	17.6	3	100
Aneurysm	11	2	18.2	2	100
Radiation arteritis	16	6	37.5	2	33.3
Takayasu's arteritis	19	5	26.3	0	—
Embolism	2	2	100	1	50.0
Total	131	30	22.9	10	33.3

TABLE 3.4. Ocular manifestations

Amaurosis fugax		16
Unilateral persistent loss of vision		9
Complete	4	
Incomplete	5	
Bilateral ischemic retinopathy		5

incidence of 22.9%. This is not significantly different from the incidence of ocular manifestations in atherosclerotic disease of the carotid bifurcation. The incidence of ocular involvement was evenly distributed among the different types of nonatherosclerotic lesions with the exception of carotid kinking where eye involvement was less frequent. Most symptoms, especially in unilateral lesions, were thromboembolic in origin, closely mimicking those of atherosclerotic disease of the carotid bifurcation, with transient retinal ischemic attacks or strokes in a total of 25 patients (83.3%) Severe alteration of vision due to bilateral ischemic retinopathy was present in three patients with bilateral occlusions of both common and internal carotid arteries. One of these patients had a radiation arteritis while the other two had Takayasu's arteritis. In two more patients with this disease, ophthalmoscopic examination showed typical signs of chronic retinal ischemia but their vision was clinically normal.

DIAGNOSIS

Diagnosis of nonatherosclerotic lesions of the carotid artery is not different from that of atherosclerotic disease. Associated cerebral symptoms are important clues but they have been present in only one-third of our patients (Table 3.3). Although rarely found, a cervical bruit should be looked for routinely. Noninvasive hemodynamic tests have their usual limitations. We have found them extremely useful in hemodynamically significant lesions. However most are negative in the presence of small emboli-producing lesions and therefore should not constitute an end-point in the evaluation of symptomatic patients. Ultrasonic imaging has been especially useful in Takayasu's arteritis since the common carotid artery is easily accessible and usually affected by considerable thickening of the arterial wall (Figure 3.17). Angiography obviously remains the cornerstone in the work-up of these patients. Except in major lesions of the intrathoracic great vessels, intravenous digital subtraction angiography has been usually insufficient, especially in the diagnosis of fibrodysplastic or high-lying lesions of the internal carotid artery. Conventional angiography

TABLE 3.5. Surgical management

Disease	*Procedure*	*N*
Kinking	Correction	4
Fibromuscular dysplasia	Dilatation	8
Dissection-aneurysm	Venous grafting	5
Radiation arteritis	Bypass from	
Takayasu's arteritis	Ascending aorta	4
	Subclavian artery	5
	to	
	Internal carotid A.	7
	Common carotid A.	2
Embolism	Embolectomy	2

or intraarterial digital subtraction angiography is necessary in most cases, both for diagnosis and proper planning of their surgical treatment.

SURGICAL MANAGEMENT

Nonatherosclerotic lesions of the carotid artery should be surgically treated when symptomatic and accessible. In asymptomatic patients surgical treatment is not justified, except in aneurysms and high-grade stenosis. Surgical management is somewhat more difficult than that of atherosclerotic lesions and may necessitate a wide variety of operative procedures (Table 3.5).

Proximal lesions affecting the common carotid arteries are reconstructed using bypass proceeding from the ascending aorta or subclavian artery, depending on the the extent of the lesion and general condition of the patient. Outflow may be limited to one or both external carotid arteries in the presence of common and internal carotid artery occlusion. However isolated reconstruction of the external carotid artery is appropriate in cases with ocular symptoms secondary to severe hypoperfusion. In such cases subtraction angiography is often necessary in order to disclose the patency of the external carotid artery and make sure that it plays a rôle in ocular vascularization.

Distal lesions affecting the carotid bifurcation or internal carotid artery are usually best treated by saphenous vein grafting. Possible exceptions may be kinking and fibromuscular dysplasia which may be treated using plastic operations and intraluminal dilatation respectively, provided major alterations of the arterial wall are not present. Embolectomy using a Fogarty catheter may also prove feasible in appropriate

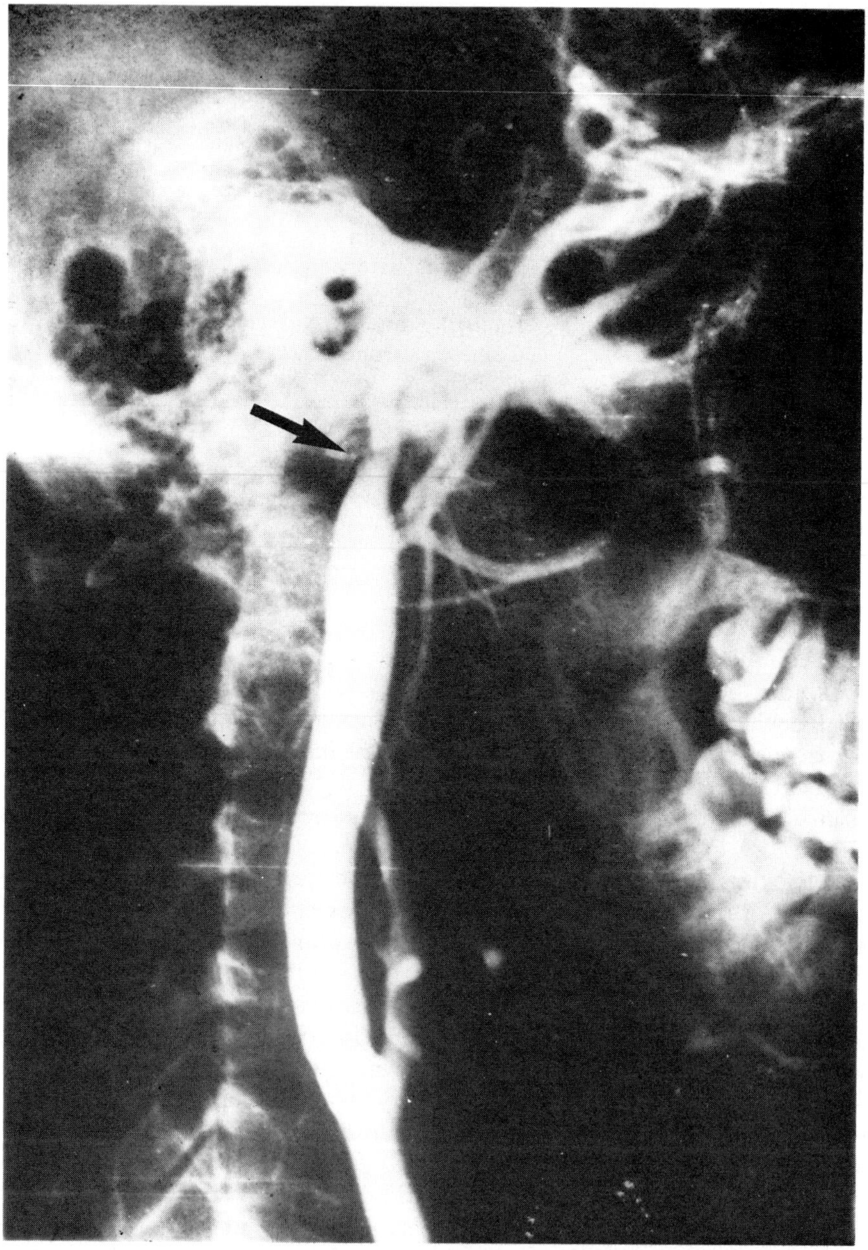

Fig. 3.19. Postoperative arteriogram showing an internal carotid replacement by a patent venous graft done through a combined cervical and intrapetrous approach. Arrow points to the distal anastomosis.

cases. A difficult technical problem concerns aneurysms of the distal extracranial internal carotid artery. Venous grafting is possible using an extended cervical approach up to the C1 level. However it remains a rather difficult procedure and the last centimeter of the artery before the bony canal is often impossible to reach. In such cases the usual alternative has been carotid ligation, either isolated (9, 16) or in combination with extracranial-intracranial bypass (1). However this probably does not constitute an optimal solution, especially in patients with bilateral lesions. Using a team-approach with ENT surgeons we have approached the intrapetrous portion of the internal carotid artery directly in a few selected cases. Although vascular results have been gratifying (Figure 3.19) the magnitude of the procedure and its attendant sequelae have discouraged us from using it more frequently. We would still consider such an approach unilaterally in the presence of bilateral lesions.

Among the entire series of 30 patients with ocular manifestations of nonatherosclerotic disease of the carotid artery there have been no postoperative deaths. One stroke occurred from occlusion of a venous graft of the internal carotid artery inserted through an extended cervical approach with technical difficulties due to poor operative exposure. In retrospect this patient should have had either simple ligation or intrapetrous surgery. Satisfying clinical and angiographic results have been obtained in all the other patients. Ischemic retinopathy has been cured completely in one patient and partially reversed in four others.

CONCLUSIONS

(a) Nonatherosclerotic disease of the carotid artery accounts for more than 10 percent of all carotid operations.
(b) The frequency of ocular manifestations is quite similar to that found in atherosclerotic lesions.
(c) Both thromboembolic and hemodynamic phenomena may be encountered.
(d) Surgical management is often complex but provides gratifying results.

REFERENCES

1. Perdue, G.D., Barreca, J.P., Smith, R.B., and King, O.W.: The significance of elongation and angulation of the carotid artery: a negative view. *Surgery* 77:45, 1975.
2. Desai, B., Toole, J.F.: Kinks, coils, and carotids: a review. *Stroke* 6:649, 1975.
3. Stanton, P.E., Jr., McClusky, D.A., and Lamis, P.A.: Hemodynamic assessment and surgical correction of kinking of the internal carotid artery. *Surgery* 84:793, 1978.

4. Vannix, R.S., Joergenson, E.J., and Carter, R.: Kinking of the internal carotid artery. *Am. J. Surg.* 134:82, 1977.
5. Effeney, D.J., Ehrenfeld, W.K., Stoney, R.J., and Wylie, E.J.: Why operate on carotid fibromuscular dysplasia? *Arch. Surg.* 115:1261, 1980.
6. Stanley, J.C., Fry, W.J., Seeger, J.F., Hoffman, G.L. and Gabrielsen, T.O.: Extracranial internal carotid and vertebral artery fibrodysplasia. *Arch. Surg.* 109:215, 1974.
7. Balaji, M.R., DeWeese, J.A.: Fibromuscular dysplasia of the internal carotid artery. *Arch. Surg.* 115:984, 1980.
8. Ehrenfeld, W.K., Wylie, E.J.: Spontaneous dissection of the internal carotid artery. *Arch. Surg.* 11:1294, 1976.
9. Busuttil, R.W., Davidson, R.K., Foley, K.T., Livesay, J.T. and Barker, W.F.: Selective management of extracranial carotid arterial aneurysms. *Am. J. Surg.* 140:85, 1980.
10. McCollum, C.H., Wheeler, W.G., Noon, G.P. and DeBakey, M.E.: Aneurysms of the extracranial carotid artery. *Am. J. Surg.* 137:196, 1979.
11. Mokri, B., Piepgras, D.G., Sundt, T.M., and Pearson, B.W.: Extracranial internal carotid artery aneurysm. *Mayo Clin. Proc.* 57:310, 1982.
12. Rhodes, E.L., Stanley, J.C., Hoffman, G.L., Gronrnwett, J.L. and Fry, W.J.: Aneurysms of extracranial carotid arteries. *Arch. Surg.* 111:339, 1976.
13. Elerding, S.C., Fernandez, R.N., Grotta, J.C., Lindberg, R.D., Causay, L.C., and McMurtrey, M.J.: Carotid artery disease following external cervical irradiation. *Ann. Surg.* 194:609, 1981.
14. Kieffer, E., Natali, J.: Supraaortic trunk lesions in Takayasu's arteritis. From Bergan, J.J., Yao, J.S.T. (Eds.) *Cerebrovascular Insufficiency*, New York: Grune & Stratton, Inc., 1983.
15. Ishilkawa, K., Uyama, M., and Asayama, K.: Occlusive thromboaortopathy (Takayasu's disease): cervical arterial stenoses, retinal arterial pressure, retinal microaneurysms and prognosis. *Stroke* 14:730, 1983.
16. Ehrenfeld, W.K., Stoney, R.J., and Wylie, E.J.: Relation of carotid stump pressure to safety of carotid artery ligation. *Surgery* 93:299, 1983.
17. Ausman, J.I., Pearce, J.E., de los Reyes, R.A. and Schanz, G.: Treatment of a high extracranial carotid aneurysm with CCA-MCA bypass and carotid ligation. *J. Neurosurg.* 58:421, 1983.

DISCUSSION: SESSION ONE

ASYMPTOMATIC HOLLENHORST PLAQUE

The panel discussed the proper work-up for an asymptomatic Hollenhorst plaque. Their consensus was that this finding indicates the need for a four-vessel arteriogram. Furthermore, if an appropriate carotid lesion is found, a carotid endarterectomy should be recommended. Feldman stressed that when they were explored even those patients with retinal emboli who showed small and smooth plaques in their arteriogram, had significant lesions in their carotids—significant in the sense that a source for the embolus, namely an ulceration or an excrescence, was demonstrated at operation. Although arteriography is still the gold standard, it is by no means infallible and on occasions ultrasound images of the carotid bifurcation reveal lesions not seen in the arteriogram.

ROLE OF INTRAVENOUS DIGITAL ARTERIOGRAPHY

The advantages of intravenous digital arteriography are obvious, but there is some doubt that the information provided by this technique is adequate to exclude ulceration in a nonstenosing plaque in patients with TIAs. Kieffer stated that even standard arteriograms are not always capable of showing ulcerated lesions that are found later at operation, let alone intravenous digital arteriograms which have considerably less resolution and are therefore inadequate for this purpose. He added that in these cases noninvasive ultrasound imaging of the carotid bifurcation often provides more information on the condition of the carotid bifurcation than a standard angiogram.

TAKAYASU'S DISEASE

The large number of paitents with Takayasu's disease reported by Kieffer aroused the interest of American surgeons who see considerably fewer cases of this entity. He was questioned as to the ethnic origin of these patients. Kieffer said that approximately two-thirds of his cases come from North Africa or the West Indies, but that 15% of those patients are natives of France.

DO ARTERIAL STENOSES PROTECT DISTAL VESSELS?

Since as the distal arteries of a kidney with a severe stenosis of its main renal artery are histologically more normal than those of the other which since has subjected to hypertension, can one say whether a carotid stenosis some way protects the intracranial circulation distal to the stenosis from atherosclerosis? In Henkind's opinion this question cannot yet be answered. He said, however, that since the complications of a carotid lesion are well known and the evidence of its presumably protective role is lacking, the strategy of operating on these lesions is probably correct.

CHANGES IN EYE NEOVASCULARIZATION WITH BYPASS OPERATIONS

Siekert was asked to expand on why his resolution of the neovascularization of the eye occurs following extraintracranial bypass. Although Siekert has observed it, he did not know how common it was or what physiological mechanism was responsible for it.

CAN ONE AVOID ARTERIOGRAMS BEFORE CAROTID OPERATIONS?

At present the morbidity of conventional arteriography is similar to that reported for carotid endarterectomy in some series. Can one avoid the risk of arteriography in a patient who has a severe carotid stenosis demonstrated by ultrasound and a normal CT scan of the brain?

The panel's opinion was that, in addition to having information about the lesion itself, one needs an arteriogram to know what the intracranial circulation looks like before deciding on an operation. Otherwise intracranial lesions of which one was not aware may go undetected even by the CT scan. Members of the panel had experience with patients sent to them for carotid endarterectomy where the noninvasive work-up had shown a lesion in the carotid which was either grossly misinterpreted or not even present when a standard arteriogram was done.

Rob recalled that years ago arteriography used to carry a much higher risk, and carotid endarterectomy was sometimes done in symptomatic patients with carotid bruits without arteriograms. He added that today, the risk of arteriography is considerably less than it was reported to be 50–60% when these alternatives were considered. Rob also related his experience with three patients, all of whom had a brain hemangioma not suspected before the operation. One of them died because of the failure to indentify the problem lesion before the operation.

CLOSED TRAUMA TO CAROTID

An audience member asked what experience there had been with closed trauma to the carotid artery in boxing and in people who overstretch their necks in an accident, thus injuring a carotid artery and suffering stroke or death. In the opinion of the panel, most patients with closed trauma to the carotid had had motorcycle rather than boxing accidents. A member of the panel related the case of a patient who injured his neck when a rope under tension broke and wrapped around his neck, causing a traumatic thrombosis of the carotid artery and hemiplegia.

ISCHEMIA FROM POSITIONAL CHANGES

Kieffer was asked how arterial obstruction resulting in symptoms could be caused by changes in head position. He answered that when there is lengthening of an artery, either congenital or because of elongation of the aortic arch due to hypertension, the vessel may kink in extreme positions of the head and neck. This is particularly common for the vertebral artery. He pointed out, however, that the subject being discussed at the meeting was focal ischemia of the eye and that entity was probably embolic in the majority of cases. He had seen hypoperfusion syndromes, such as vertebrobasilar insufficiency, from positional kinking of arteries but had never seen it cause retinal ischemia.

Rob was asked to expand on his statement that mental slowing may be an indication to operate on a carotid stenosis in an otherwise asymptomatic patient. He said that he had done psychometric testing before and after operation in patients who had severe occlusive disease of the cerebral blood supply and had shown that there was considerable improvement of test scores following revascularization. He restated that some of the so-called asymptomatic patients who suffer mental deterioration are in fact showing symptoms of reduction of cerebral blood flow and should be considered symptomatic.

TRANSTEMPORAL INTERNAL CAROTID RECONSTRUCTION

Regarding his technique for reconstruction of the internal carotid at the base of the skull, Kieffer mentioned that he is at present very disenchanted with the procedure. The technique involves cutting through the temporal bone and is accompanied by the appearance of serious neurological and audiological deficits.

II

THE EYE

4

THE CLINICAL SIGNIFICANCE OF RETINAL EMBOLI

R.W. Ross Russell, M.D.

In the retinal circulation, which shares a common origin with the cerebral circulation, the identification of an arterial embolus may be a valuable indication of vascular or cardiac disease. The varied behavior of retinal emboli, deduced either from direct observation or from fluorescein angiography provides a unique insight into the pathological, vascular reactions of the retinal microcirculation. The appearance, clinical effects, and management of the main types of retinal emboli are reviewed. The causes of reduced ocular blood flow are outlined in Table 4.1.

RETINAL PLATELET EMBOLI

Numerous reports have appeared of patients with brief episodes of unilateral amaurosis fugax in whom white bodies have been observed to pass along the retinal arteries during the period of visual loss (1). The appearance of the white bodies has varied a little from patient to patient, probably reflecting a difference in the volume of embolic material. Some reports describe small white plugs moving rapidly from bifurcation to bifurcation, tending to pause at each, sometimes breaking into smaller fragments and eventually disappearing completely in the peripheral arterioles (2). The whole process usually takes a few minutes.

In other reports the white segment has been larger and has moved more sluggishly, behaving as a viscid liquid flowing slowly through the major retinal arteries (3).

From the National Hospital for Nervous Diseases, St. Thomas' Hospital, and Moorfields Eye Hospital, London, England

TABLE 4.1. Causes of reduced ocular blood flow

Microembolism	*Reduced perfusion pressure*	*Increased retinal vascular resistance*
Carotid artery atheroma	Severe bilateral atheroma	Hypertension
Cardiac valvular disease	Aortic arch syndrome	Diabetes
	Carotid-cavernous fistula	Polycythemia
	Glaucoma	Dysproteinemia
	Raised intracranial pressure	? spasm

Obviously no pathological examination has been made of such transient and trivial phenomena. It seems very likely, however, that these are emboli, largely composed of aggregated platelets. The evidence for this may be summarized as follows:

(a) The physical characteristics and in vivo behavior of verified platelet thrombi in animals corresponds closely to those observed in the human retina (4).
(b) Mural thrombi of mixed platelet and fibrin composition are frequently found in the internal carotid artery in patients with amaurosis fugax who have undergone carotid endarterectomy (5).
(c) In two patients who died following carotid thrombosis, platelet aggregates were confirmed histologically in the ophthalmic and retinal arteries (2,3).
(d) Patients with very frequent attacks of amaurosis fugax often show qualitative platelet defects such as an increased platelet turnover or an increased tendency to aggregation (6). Such patients may also show a dramatic response to aspirin therapy (7).
(e) Similar white retinal emboli have been described in patients with platelet disorders such as thrombocythemia (8).

Because the attacks are so brief, the chance of actually viewing an embolism is small and it is not possible to estimate accurately what proportion of patients with amaurosis fugax are experiencing attacks of this type. The following clinical characteristics point toward platelet embolism as the responsible mechanism in an individual patient: very frequent attacks, normal retinal appearances between attacks, absence of permanent signs of retinal ischemia or of visual field defect.

The source of platelet emboli is most commonly fresh thrombus in the internal carotid artery usually originating in the carotid sinus but sometimes propagating throughout the vessel. Other possible sources include the cardiac valves in chronic rheumatic heart disease and occasionally in acute rheumatic fever. Platelet thrombi have also been reported in prosthetic heart valves, mitral valve leaflet prolapse, carotid dissection or trauma, fibromuscular dysplasia or carotid arteritis (9,10).

CHOLESTEROL EMBOLI

In patients with advanced atherosclerosis of the aorta or large vessels the intimal plaques may ulcerate, thus exposing the contents of the lesions to the blood stream. Cholesterol containing material may then be swept off to embolize in small distal arteries. This has been shown to occur in the arteries of the leg, kidney, and intestines (11). The cerebral and ocular circulations are less severely affected since ulcerating atheroma does not often spread to the ascending aorta or aortic arch. However, when atheroma affects the carotid arteries, cholesterol emboli may be carried to the retina or brain. The chemical composition of the retinal emboli in these cases has been shown to correspond closely to that of the atheromatous lesion in the carotid artery (12).

Such patients are usually middle-aged or elderly males with a high prevalence of arterial risk factors, such as hypertension, diabetes, and hypercholesterolemia.

Cholesterol emboli have a highly characteristic appearance in the retinal circulation. They are small, often multiple, shiny yellow plaques lodged in the retinal branch arteries, usually on the temporal side of the disc (13). The site of the impaction is usually, but not invariably, at a bifurcation. Sometimes a shower of small emboli may lodge simultaneously in many branch arterioles around the macula.

Some, but not all, cholesterol emboli cause a significant obstruction to blood flow. The degree of obstruction depends upon the angle at which the flat crystalline structure is impacted (10). They have a tendency to move distally in the course of a few days and usually disappear entirely over a three month period. Regions of retinal cloudy swelling or cotton wool spots may be present in relation to the blocked vessel and there are occasionally small amounts of retinal hemorrhage.

Patients with cholesterol emboli usually present with amaurosis fugax, but emboli of this kind may also be seen in symptomless patients. It is common to find no evidence of retinal ischemia or field defect. On some occasions, however, altitudinal or sectorial defects may be present, corresponding to areas of retinal ischemia, and when multiple macular emboli are present there may be a central scotoma.

At the time of examination the degree of field loss may be disproportionately severe when compared to the size and number of emboli. This is explained by movement of emboli in the intervening period.

A highly characteristic feature of cholesterol emboli is the localized sheathing reaction which develops in retinal arteries at the point of impaction. This represents a giant cell foreign body reaction to the cholesterol crystal lodged in the wall (14). The reactions persist for months or years afterwards, but probably not indefinitely. The finding of localized sheathing reaction has the same clinical significance as cholesterol embolism.

Cholesterol emboli are the commonest type of emboli found in the retina. They comprised 87% in a recent published series (15). Although often causing trivial or short-lived visual loss, they are important in indicating an ulcerated atherosclerotic lesion in a proximal artery which may be the source of further thromboembolism to the brain. There is a strong association with stenosis of the internal carotid artery. Other emboli may originate in the aorta, but cholesterol emboli probably do not arise from the heart itself.

No medical treatment appears likely to influence cholesterol embolism. If the source can be identified it may be possible to remove the atheromatous ulcer by surgical endarterectomy. This is the treatment of choice of those patients with accessible and localized lesions in the internal carotid artery. Patients who appear on grounds of age and vascular status to be fit for arterial surgery, should be investigated by carotid angiography or digital subtraction angiography.

THROMBOTIC EMBOLI

The proportions of fibrin, platelets and erythrocytes found in intravascular thrombus appear to depend principally on the physical characteristics of blood flow prevailing at the time of formation. Thrombus formed in rapidly flowing blood, as in an artery, tends to be composed of intact, aggregated platelets. As these fuse and lose their granules increasing amounts of fibrin may be identified as strands between the clumps of platelets. These stabilize the platelet plug making it less likely to embolize. Thrombin, as well as initiating coagulation, acts as a potent platelet aggregating agent, and the two main components of thrombus, platelet clumps, and fibrin strands, are formed concurrently. When there is partial or complete stagnation of flow, or when thrombosis takes place in slowly moving blood as in the large veins, large numbers of red cells become enmeshed in the fibrin network.

Thrombotic emboli to the retinal circulation are unusual. Probably they are too large to enter the ophthalmic artery and tend instead to impact at the carotid bifurcation or in the middle cerebral artery. In the retinal arteries they appear as white or dark red segments, completely obstructing blood flow over a length of retinal artery and producing cloudy swelling of the nerve fiber layer. Fluorescein angiography confirms the obstruction and usually indicates survival of the capillary bed. Patients present with one or more episodes of visual loss, usually of a nerve fiber type and often permanent. The prognosis for recovery depends on the duration of occlusion. Small emboli may disappear entirely in a few days, presumably under the action of natural fibrinolysis. The micro-circulation then returns to normal. In other patients the occlusion lasts longer. Organization and recannalization of the thrombotic segment takes place, producing a length of sheathed and attenuated retinal artery (11). In these cases the visual field defect is permanent.

Retinal emboli of this type usually originate from the cavities of the heart in patients with chronic rheumatic heart disease, ischemic heart disease, or occasionally from the venous side of the circulation through patent septum. Long term anticoagulation is the treatment of choice.

CALCIFIC EMBOLI

Calcific emboli comprise only 4% of the emboli found in the retina (15). The embolus is single, white, chalky in appearance, and lodges permanently in the retinal arteries. It tends to block completely one of the upper or lower branches and to produce an appropriate arcuate or sectorial defect. It may also lodge at the lamina cribrosa. A characteristic feature is the formation of collateral vessels to bypass the occluded segment of vessel which is eventually reduced to a white bloodless cord. The source of these emboli is invariably the cardiac valves, either aortic or mitral (11). The patients usually suffer from chronic rheumatic heart disease. It is advisable to undertake a full cardiac assessment in these patients, since the occurrence of a retinal embolus is sometimes an indication that the valve is crumbling and may require surgical replacement in the near future.

RARE TYPES OF EMBOLI

There are a number of rare types of retinal emboli (16). These include tumor emboli (usually atrial myxoma), fat emboli following fracture of a long bone, septic emboli during subacute bacterial endocarditis (these are very small and usually produce multiple hemorrhages). Talc emboli may occur in drug abusers, and silicone emboli to the retina have followed injections of cosmetic materials into the face or scalp.

REFERENCES

1. Fisher, C.M.: Observations of the fundus oculi in transient monocular blindness. *Neurology* 9:333, 1959.
2. Russell, R.W.R.: Observations on the retinal blood vessels in monocular blindness. *Lancet* ii:1422, 1961.
3. McBrien, D.J., Bradley, R.D. and Ashton, N.: The nature of retinal emboli in stenosis of the internal carotid artery. *Lancet* i:697, 1963.
4. Honour, A.J., Russell, R.W.R.: Experimental platelet embolism. *Brit. J. Exp. Pathol.* 43:350, 1962.
5. Gunning, A.J., Pickering, G.W., Robb-Smith, A.H.T., and Russell, R.W.R.: Mural thrombosis of the internal carotid artery and subsequent embolism. *Quart. J. Med.* 33:155, 1964.
6. Wilson, L.A.: Platelet survival in amaurosis fugax. In Breddin, K., Dorndorf, W., Leow, D., and Marx, R. eds.: *Fourth Calfarit-Symposium, Berlin.* Stuttgart: Schatteur Verlag, 1977.
7. Harrison, M.J.G., Marshall, J., Meadows, J.C., and Russell, R.W.R.: The effect of aspirin in amaurosis fugax. *Lancet* ii:743, 1971.
8. Davies-Jones, G.A.B., Preston, F.E., and Timperley, W.R.: *Neurological complications in clinical haematology.* Oxford: Blackwell, 1980.
9. Barnett, H.J.M., Baughner, D.R., Taylor, D.W., Cooper, P.E., Kostak, W. and Nichol, P.M.: Further evidence relating to mitral valve prolapse in cerebral ischemic events. *N. Eng. J. Med.* 302:139, 1980.
10. Russell, R.W.R.: The source of retinal emboli. *Lancet* ii:789, 1968.
11. Holley, K.E., Bahn, R.C., McGoon, D.C., and Mankin, H.T.: Calcific embolization associated with valvotomy for calcific aortic stenosis. *Circulation* 28:175, 1963.
12. David, N.J., Klintworth, G.K., Friedberg, S.J., and Dillon, M.: Fatal atheromatous cerebral embolism associated with bright plaques in the retinal arterioles. Report of a case. *Neurology*, 13:708, 1963.
13. Hollenhorst, R.W.: Significance of bright plaques in the retinal arterioles. *J.A.M.A.* 178:23, 1961.
14. Dark, A.J., Rizk, S.N.: Progressive focal sclerosis of retinal arteries: a sequel to impaction of cholesterol emboli. *Brit. Med. J.* 1:270, 1967.
15. Arruga, J., Sanders, M.D.: Ophthalmologic findings in 70 patients with evidence of retinal embolism. *Ophthalmology* 89:1336, 1982.
16. Russell, R.W.R.: Less common varieties of cerebral arterial disease. In Russell, R.W.R. ed: *Vascular Disease of the Central Nervous System.* New York: Churchill Livingstone, 1983.
17. Zimmerman, L.E.: Embolism of central retinal artery secondary to myocardial infarction with mural thrombosis. *Arch. Ophthalmol.* 73:822, 1965.

5

THE EYE AS A CAROTID TRANSDUCER; THE TRANSDUCER AS A CAROTID EYE

Roger F. Higgins, Ph.D.

This chapter addresses noninvasive assessment of the carotid bifurcation as a source of embolic material seen in the circulation of the eye and as a cause for the manifestations of postocular ischemia such as ischemic optic neuritis. It considers as well, the noninvasive evaluation of asymptomatic carotid disease.

There are two parts to this chapter. The first concerns the use of real-time high resolution B-mode ultrasonic imaging as a carotid bifurcation scanning technique. Another section considers the use of oculoplethysmography (OPG-Gee) to assess the hemodynamic significance of stenotic lesions in the common and internal carotid arteries, that is, determining whether the stenotic lesion significantly impairs volume flow rate or causes a significant pressure gradient to form with corresponding distal hypotension.

REAL-TIME B-MODE IMAGING—THE TRANSDUCER AS A CAROTID EYE

Current state-of-the-art real-time B-mode carotid bifurcation imagers are capable of displaying sections of soft tissue approximately 4 cm deep by 3 cm wide, the plane of the section being determined by the precise orientation of the transducer head. The image display is of the video type and may contain as many as 256 grey scale increments. The human eye has the ability to discern only a small fraction of this number of grey scales,

From the Vascular Surgery Laboratory, Harper-Grace Hospitals, Detroit, Michigan.

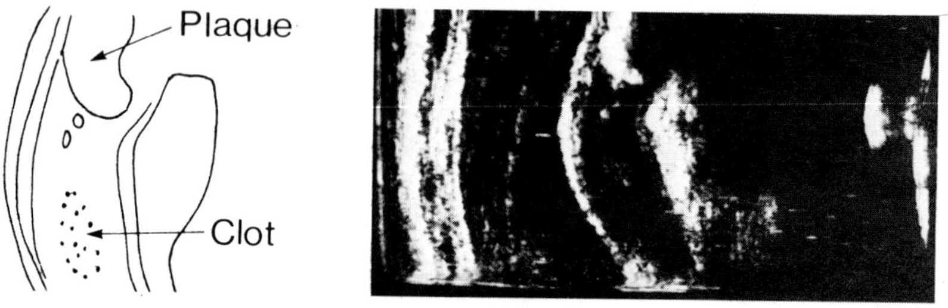

Fig. 5.1. Posterior lateral view of the right common carotid proximal to the carotid bulb. (Patient's head is toward the top of the picture.) Densely calcified plaque is seen at uppermost part of image. Lesion restricted flow to point where clot could form in proximal common carotid. Clot is visible in this "still" picture but its real size and consistency are misrepresented.

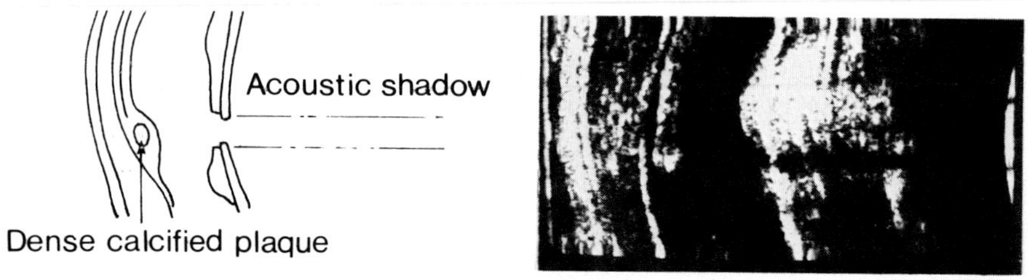

Fig. 5.2. Anterior view of left carotid bulb (patient's head is to bottom of picture) showing area of dense calcification in anterior wall. Variety of approach angles may be necessary to avoid calcified plaque in near field in order to demonstrate far field detail.

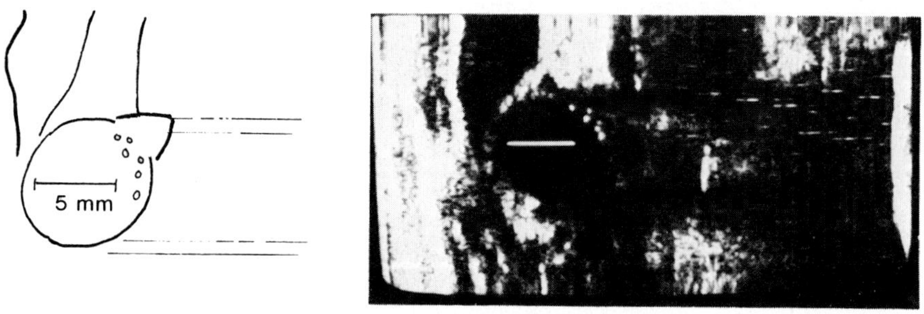

Fig. 5.3. Transverse view at mid-level of left common carotid artery showing left vertebral artery implanted into common carotid artery. First part of vertebral artery can be seen on upper right margin of common carotid artery.

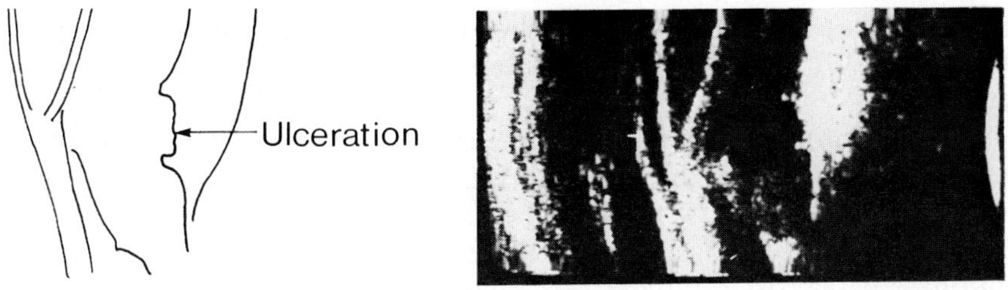

Fig. 5.4. Lateral view of the left carotid bulb showing the rim of a shallow ulceration (1 mm deep) which was not visualized by two-plane arteriography.

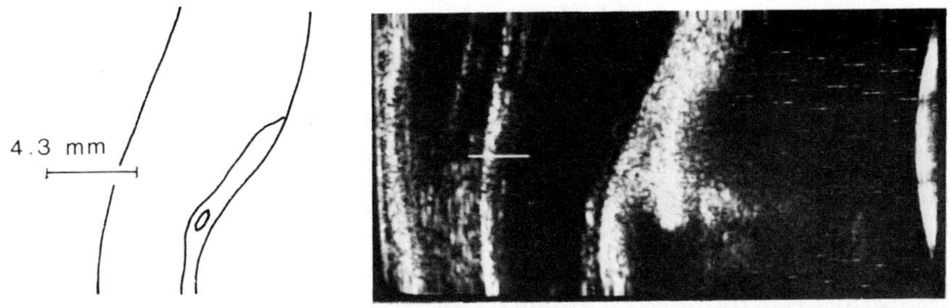

Fig. 5.5. Lateral view of left common carotid artery showing a thickened intima on the deep wall. Luminal surface of plaque suggests roughness, which may be representative of a shallow ulceration. Grey-scale manipulation might possibly help identify presence of thrombus on surface of this plaque, thereby establishing presence of ulceration.

meaning that the B-mode imager may be able to differentiate between subtle structural differences which the human eye cannot appreciate.

Many components and features of the atherosclerotic plaque may be readily recognized in the B-mode image. The density of a particular structure or substance in the image determines its grey-scale representation. Thus, dense features such as bone and calcified atherosclerotic plaque appear very bright, while blood and water, the least dense, appear as the darkest greys.

A further feature of the modality is its real-time format, whereby the video image is updated rapidly enough for the investigator to be virtually unaware of the frame-by-frame presentation of the data. Indeed, the image update rate is sufficiently rapid that one can easily appreciate moment-by-moment changes within the subject, such as the pulsatile radial movement of arterial walls in response to cardiac activity and larger changes in jugular vein size caused by respiration and swallowing. Much more subtle movements are also discernible, allowing the identification of a small intimal flap, for example, as it oscillates in a high velocity flow field during systole.

Another important attribute of the real-time image is the way it allows one to identify recent thrombus formations which are somewhat more mature than fresh clot. This thrombotic feature takes on a reciprocating, speckled, almost scintillating appearance which is markedly pronounced in real-time but almost totally unrecognizable in a single freeze-frame view (Fig 5.1) and, like other unique phenomena, must be seen to be believed. More mature thrombus is denser, thus brighter, and does not move; thus one may date an occlluded vessel as recent or old.

Resolution is to a certain extent dependent upon image composition. Dense structures tend to block the ultrasound beam with the result that detail behind the dense layer is lost in what has come to be known as an acoustic shadow (Fig. 5.2). In a more balanced image, a line of fine sutures (for example 6-0 Prolene) may easily be identified (Fig. 5.3). Irregularities of submillimeter size may be shown by a talented operator using a variety of different angles of approach to obtain an optimal view (Fig. 5.4). In this respect the B-mode imager appears to be more accurate than the arteriogram, inasmuch as it is capable of showing detail that is entirely missing in even the highest quality catheter study. This is of particular importance in the case of very small ulcerations in minimal athersclerotic plaques which may be responsible for embolic problems such as TIA's.

Strictly speaking present B-mode imagers cannot identify an ulceration, which is true roughness of the luminal surface of the artery (Fig. 5.5). There is no sure way to distinguish surface roughness and true ulceration using either B-mode imaging or arteriography. This limitation, as it applies to arteriography, has been well recognized also, in two situations. First, on many occasions the pronounced roughness seen on arteriography has turned out at operation to be a craterous plaque entirely covered with a smooth, glistening pseudo-intima, not a true ulceration. Second, other less dramatic-looking lesions on arteriography have been found to consist of leaking pockets of grumous, fatty fibrin debris slowly being extruded into the blood stream. When B-mode imaging reveals the presence of roughness on the luminal arterial surface of a small, well-defined lesion, attention should be paid to the relative density of the underlying plaque. The tissue characterization capability of B-mode imaging has allowed at least two sub-categories of luminal surface lesions to be identified, each having an effect upon interpretation and, possibly, treatment.

Ulcerations are frequently associated with earlier, less dense atherosclerosis, thus luminal irregularities in association with less dense plaque are more likely to be true ulcerations (Fig. 5.6). Conversely, rough surfaces on dense calcified plaques (Fig. 5.7) are sometimes covered with pseudointima, are less likely to contain ulcerations, and may, therefore, represent a less volatile stage of the disease.

A good proportion of atherosclerotic lesions, however, contain both hard and soft zones (Fig. 5.8), roughness and ulceration, constituting what is quite accurately described as complicated plaque.

The problem of differentiating true ulceration from the more benign roughness would be easier if there was a greater grey-scale differentiation between normal blood and fresh clot. The density, and thus the echogenic characteristics, of moving blood and fresh clot are very similar, and the reflected signals from each are represented as dark shades very close together on the grey scale. A solution to this problem must await a new generation of imagers that will allow more grey scale manipulation than is currently feasible.

Occasionally, a smooth, soft finger of plaque will be seen extending far into the bloodstream (Fig. 5.9). The appearance and motion of such lesions are a powerful stimulus to take action even in the absence of vessel wall roughness.

In chapter 2 of this text, Dr. Feldman has amply dealt with the broad range of symptomatic carotid lesions. He notes that lesions responsible for ocular symptoms span the entire range of the atherosclerotic disease process, from very small ulcerations in minimal plaque (see Fig. 5.4) to total internal carotid artery occlusions (see Fig. 5.1). In the last decade a variety of noninvasive methods have been proposed to identify carotid bifurcation disease, usually as the underlying cause of an asymptomatic carotid bruit. But since the vast majority of such tests are sensitive to hemodynamic changes within the blood flow field, rather than morphological changes within the vessel wall, the arteriogram has remained the definitive way to rule out ulcerative lesions of the carotid bifurcation.

The fact that an arteriogram tends to underestimate the true extent of disease notwithstanding, it has become the "gold standard" against which all other tests are compared. Only recently has the purity of this gold standard been questioned and there is now mounting evidence that real-time B-mode imaging is a more accurate way than arteriography of examining the carotid bifurcations for embolizing ulcerations. It might seem from this that the B-mode image would shortly surplant the arteriogram as the purer standard. After considering other features of the arteriogram which the B-mode image cannot and probably never will provide, one may conclude that this will not necessarily transpire.

For example, intracerebral arteriographic views provide information about concomitant vascular disease, such as intracranial berry aneurysms, arteriovenous malformations and stenosis of the cerebral arteries and distal internal carotid arteries at the level of the carotid syphon, any of which may be responsible for the symptoms under investigation. Space-occupying

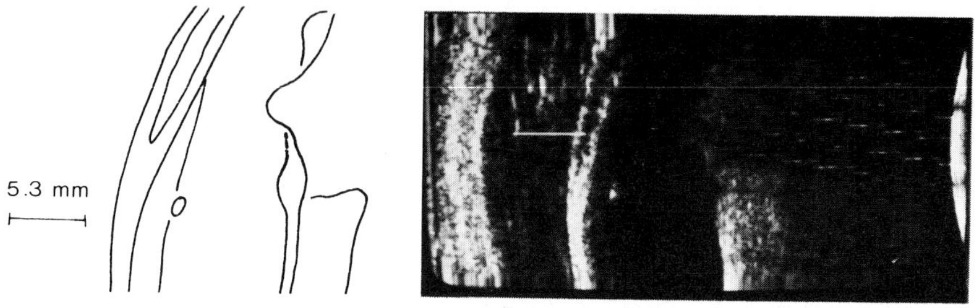

Fig. 5.6. Posterolateral view of origin of right internal carotid artery showing very subtle grey-scale changes associated with true ulceration containing fresh clot and cholesterol fragments. Lesion consisted of ruptured sac containing soft, grumous material at the time of carotid endarterectomy.

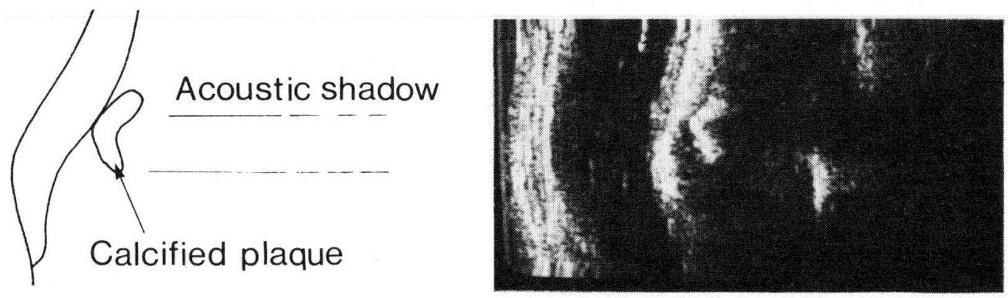

Fig. 5.7. Lateral view of left carotid bulb showing a bright, calcified plaque. The luminal surface of this lesion appears to contain a deep crater.

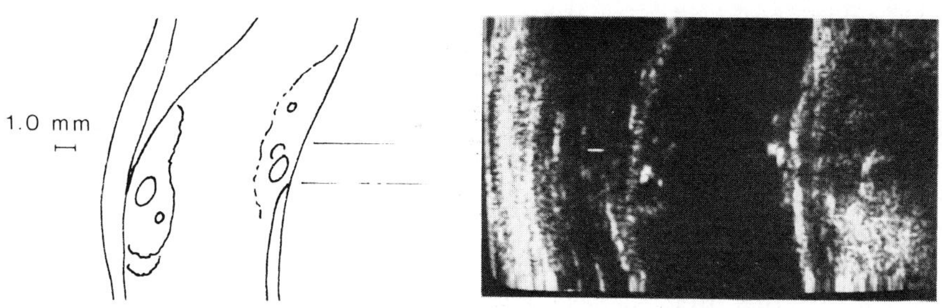

Fig. 5.8. Anterior view of the right carotid bulb showing plaque of mixed composition containing both hard and soft constituents. Luminal roughness is also present. Dense fragments separated from the vessel wall by dark band may represent plaque pushed into vessel lumen by intramural hemorrhage, a condition which must be acted upon immediately.

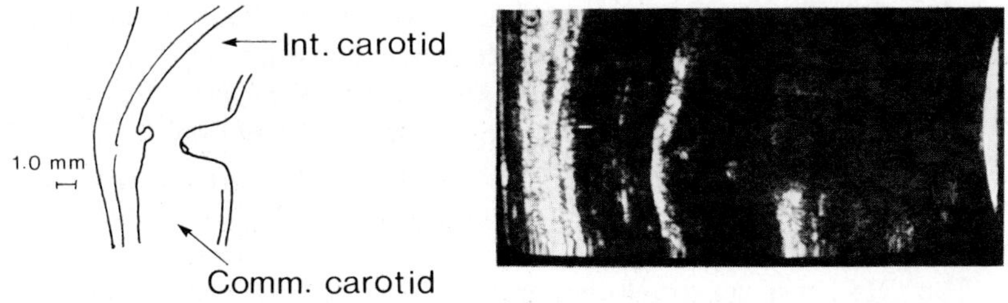

Fig. 5.9. Lateral view of right carotid bulb and the origin of the right internal carotid artery showing finger of soft plaque. In Real-time this plaque clearly waves back and forth during the systolic phase of flow. Plaque of mixed composition is present on anterior wall of artery and some luminal irregularity can be seen.

lesions such as brain tumors may present with TIA-like symptoms and must be taken into consideration when interpreting the arteriogram.

At present there is an understandable reluctance to proceed to operation on the basis of real-time B-mode information alone. A crucial question to be answered is, "In patients with classic TIA symptoms and carotid bifurcation lesions, well-defined by B-mode imaging, how many have more distal concomitant lesions that contraindicate carotid endarterectomy?" While an informal survey may put the rate at very low, that is not the same as nil.

A small (less than 10%) but significant portion of B-mode studies are not useful because they fail to adequately reveal the vessels of the carotid bifurcation, either because the vessels are too deep or because the bifurcation is too high under the mandible.

OCULOPLETHYSMOGRAPHIC ASSESSMENT OF THE ASYMPTOMATIC CAROTID BRUIT—THE EYE AS A CAROTID TRANSDUCER

In oculoplethysmographic (OPG [Gee]) assessment of the asymptomatic carotid bruit, the eye acts as a "carotid transducer." Important as this subject is as a mainstay of noninvasive vascular testing, its significance is lessened considerably in the presence of eye pathology. Those patients who are directed by their opthalmologist to a vascular laboratory are very likely to be symptomatic (whether they are aware of it or not) and, in accordance with prevailing wisdom, will ultimately be recommended for arteriography instead of OPG (Gee) testing. This is true for two reasons: (a) OPG (Gee) testing is only truly positive in cases of high-grade, hemodynamically significant, uncompensated lesions. This severe condition is too far toward the late stage of the disease spectrum to try to apply to the many patients with eye symptoms possibly originating from hemodynamically insignificant plaques. (b) A compromised blood supply to the back of the eye, particularly if involving the choroid or ophthalmic arteries, may result in a false positive OPG (Gee) study. The explanation for this lies in an understanding of what it is that an OPG (Gee) test measures.

The OPG test, as developed and documented by William Gee, hence OPG (Gee), determines the systolic pressure in the ophthalmic artery using the eye globe as a pressure source, in much the same way a blood pressure cuff determines the brachial systolic pressure. As pressure in the cuff is reduced it ceases to overcome systolic pressure and the first arterial sound is heard through the stethoscope. In OPG (Gee) testing the intraocular pressure is raised by applying a suction cup to the lateral sclera of each eye with a vacuum of 500 mmHg. The evacuated suction cup distorts the eye globe causing the intraocular pressure to rise. A vacuum pressure of 500 mmHg causes a 145 mmHg intraocular pressure. As the vacuum is reduced, the intraocular pressure falls. At the point where the eye globe begins to pulsate with cardiac frequency, the pressure in the globe no longer exceeds systolic pressure in the ophthalmic artery. An OPG(Gee) unit very accurately records eye pulsations, applied vacuum, and an ECG signal, which together allow a determination of ophthalmic artery systolic pressure to be made with confidence. Clearly, confidence will be sharply reduced in cases where the posterior chamber of the eye manifests changes associated with widespread ischemia.

Small cholesterol crystals commonly seen in individual retinal arteries are responsible for insignificant changes in the total eye inflow figure and thus would not, by themselves, be likely to produce false positive OPG results.

Of equal concern are false negative OPG(Gee) studies, i.e., if the test fails to identify a major loss of luminal or cross-sectional area at the proximal end of the internal carotid artery when such is present. A major loss might be as much as 90%, although a 75% loss of area is widely considered a realistic threshold for a positive OPG(Gee) result to be obtained. One explanation for a false negative OPG(Gee) test is the possibility of a "compensated" lesion, wherein the reduction in flow caused by a very high-grade stenosis at the origin of the internal carotid artery is adequately compensated for distally by collateral circuits such as the external carotid artery connections about the eye and the Circle of Willis.

Conversely, an "uncompensated" lesion in the primary arterial pathway exists when collateral circulation fails to restore inflow deficits produced by that lesion. Inadequate compensation for a hemodynamically significant proximal arterial lesion results in distal hypotension and a measurable systolic pressure gradient between the ophthalmic arteries. Ophthalmic systolic pressure gradients in excess of 5 mmHg measured by the OPG(Gee) technique in the asymptomatic patient are reliably associated with an uncompensated, or hemodynamically significant lesion somewhere in the arterial pathway between the aortic arch and the opthalmic artery. The presence of a bruit over the carotid bifurcation on the side with the lower pressure will further suggest that the test is a true positive and that the lesion is in its usual location—the proximal internal carotid artery or the distal common carotid artery.

In patients with a positive OPG(Gee) test the absence of a carotid bruit may indicate one of three situations. Two of these are extremes: either total occlusion of the common or internal carotid arteries or no significant disease in the carotid bifurcation region, a situation which can easily be clarified by B-mode imaging. A clean carotid bifurcation and a positive OPG(Gee) test suggest a lesion elsewhere in the system, perhaps at the carotid syphon or in the ophthalmic artery. Noninvasive testing can not reliably predict the true location of such lesions.

The third situation is that where the stenosis is very far advanced but the artery is not yet totally occluded. Such lesions rarely make discernible noise and are thus indistinguishable from total occlusions using OPG(Gee) and auscultation. There is, however, an important reason for wanting to make the distinction, and that is, a tightly stenosed internal carotid artery may be endarterectomized, thereby avoiding the possibility of an ischemic stroke subsequent to final thrombosis of the artery. An already occluded internal carotid artery is not ordinarily endarterectomized and the subject had either suffered the consequences (in which case very little, not even arteriography, may be offered) or the subject has been spared. It is possible, though frequently more difficult, to make the distinction between total occlusion and near total occlusion using the B-mode imager.

The fact that a subject may undergo total occlusion of one internal carotid artery completely without symptoms indicates that some of the stenotic lesions identified by noninvasive testing could be left untreated, but which ones? It is tempting to suggest, but difficult to substantiate, that it is those subjects with well-compensated lesions [false negative OPG(Gee)] who are more likely to sustain an asymptomatic internal carotid artery occlusion, with thrombus propagation being curtailed by vigorous collateral flow in the distal vessels. The converse of the above situation is equally appealing but similarly unsubstantiated. The low flow associated with hypotension distal to an uncompensated stenosis [true positive OPG(Gee)] would be insufficient to prevent thrombosis extension into the branches of the internal carotid artery, which results in the usually catastrophic changes of an acute stroke.

SUMMARY

An attempt has been made to identify the strengths and weaknesses of real-time B-mode imaging, OPG(Gee) testing, and conventional arteriography, particularly as they relate to patients with ocular manifestations of the arterial disease process, more generally all lateralizing TIAs and also asymptomatic carotid bruits. The ways in which the results of these tests may be combined to described the underlying problem and suggest a course of action are summarized:

(a) Patients with ocular symptoms of arterial disease should have the carotid bifurcations examined by B-mode imaging prior to arteriography.
(b) Younger patients with soft rough plaques in the carotid bifurcation and ipsilateral eye symptoms may not require arteriography prior to endarterectomy.
(c) Patients with completed strokes and total occlusion of the internal carotid artery may be spared arteriography if the B-mode plaque shows a mature blockage.
(d) Patients with deficits of very recent onset may benefit from emergency thromboendarterectomy if the B-mode image shows soft, young clot occluding the internal carotid artery.
(e) Soft plaque shown by B-mode imaging is considered more unstable than hard plaque.
(f) Roughness usually represents ulceration in soft plaques, as demonstrated in B-mode imaging.
(g) Roughness may or may not be an ulceration in a densely calcified plaque as identified by B-mode imaging.
(h) Any carotid plaque, rough or smooth, hard or soft, must be seriously considered as a source for embolic material in the symptomatic patient.
(i) The hemodynamic significance of a densely calcified carotid artery bifurcation may be further assessed by OPG(Gee) testing, and if OPG(Gee) is positive the likely consequences of an occlusion must be considered. If OPG(Gee) is negative the lesion may either be overstated in the B-mode image, or it is truly narrow but adequately compensated. In an elderly, frail patient one might argue that the latter lesion represents less of a threat than might a prophylactic endarterectomy.
(j) An asymptomatic carotid bruit should be assessed with an OPG(Gee) test; if positive, a prophylactic endarterectomy should be considered since the lesion is uncompensated. If negative, B-mode imaging can identify the source of the bruit (perhaps the

external carotid artery) and categorize the composition of the underlying lesion. If this in turn is found to be of the unstable type, it may merit surgical intervention or if it is more stable, frequent noninvasive followup may be appropriate.

(k) Arteriography should be reserved for prospective candidates for surgery. If the patient is an unacceptably high surgical risk or refuses to consent to surgery, an arteriogram will not be required.

(l) The above recommendations are predicated on a combined morbidity and mortality rate for arteriography and vascular reconstruction that is acceptably low.

6

CENTRAL RETINAL ARTERY OCCLUSION AND CAROTID ARTERY DISEASE

Sohan Singh Hayreh M.D., Ph.D

We conducted a prospective investigation of 61 patients (64 eyes) with central retinal artery occlusion, concentrating particularly upon the role of carotid artery disease in the production of central retinal artery occlusion and its associated complication, ocular neovascularization. A detailed account was reported elsewhere (1); the subject is reviewed briefly here.

MATERIALS AND METHODS

Our 61 patients with central retinal artery occlusion could be divided into two groups:

Central Retinal Artery Occlusion Without Ocular Neovascularization

Group I consisted of 50 patients and 52 eyes. Forty two of the 50 patients were seen by the cardiothoracic surgeons for carotid artery evaluation. In the remaining eight patients, we felt that the central retinal artery occlusion was due to fairly apparent causes unrelated to carotid artery disease, for example, temporal arteritis, severe arterial hypertension (blood pressure $\geq$200/120 mmHg), rheumatic heart disease or other cardiac disorders. All of the 42 patients underwent noninvasive studies, including Doppler studies, and 32 patients underwent aortic arch arteriography. The rest did not have angiography, either because it was not recommended by the surgeons (seven people) or because the patient refused (three people). Table 6.1 gives the angiographic findings. One patient had internal carotid artery

TABLE 6.1. Incidence of carotid artery disease, as revealed by aortic arch arteriography

	Incidence in central retinal artery occlusion	
Carotid artery disease	*With neovascularization*	*Without neovascularization*
Complete occlusion	5	1
Stenosis	1 (80% stenosis)	2 (mild stenosis)
Stenosis and plaque	2	4
Plaque only	—	12
ICA tortuous	—	2
No detectable abnormality	2*	11
Total cases investigated	10	32

*One patient had proliferative diabetic retinopathy and another one had retinal vasculitis.

occlusion on the side of central retinal artery occlusion, with abnormal findings from Doppler studies, and a carotid bruit on the other side. No carotid angiography was done in this patient, and he was the only one with abnormal findings from Doppler studies.

One patient developed central retinal artery occlusion secondary to a carotid endarterectomy that had been performed elsewhere. In three patients who refused angiography, there was evidence of carotid artery disease on the side of central retinal artery occlusion, i.e., they had experienced a cerebrovascular accident, transient ischemic attacks, or reduced carotid pulse. In the 32 patients with angiography and the five patients mentioned above, we found that 26 (70%) had definite evidence of carotid artery disease on the side of the central retinal artery occlusion. On angiography, five patients who did not have demonstrable carotid artery disease on the side of the central retinal artery occlusion, showed the presence of plaque, stenosis, or both on the other side. Thus, of 37 patients, 26 (70%) showed definite evidence of carotid artery disease on the side of the central retinal artery occlusion, and 31 (84%) showed it on one side or the other. In the remaining five patients where the thoracic surgeons did not recommend carotid arteriography because noninvasive tests gave normal results, the possibility of carotid artery lesions such as plaques, ulcers, or even minor stenosis could not be ruled out. Overall then, 26 of 50 patients (52%) in Group I showed definite evidence of carotid artery disease on the side of the central retinal artery occlusion, but the actual incidence of carotid artery disease might have been even higher had all 42 patients referred to the cardiothoracic surgeons been investigated by carotid arteriography.

Central Retinal Artery Occlusion With Ocular Neovascularization

Group II consisted of 11 patients and 12 eyes: In this group aortic arch arteriography was performed in 10 patients. One patient refused angiography but showed a pattern of ocular disease similar to that seen in other patients with neovascular glaucoma and, hence, this patient has been included. Of the two patients with no detectable abnormality on carotid arteriography, one had long-standing juvenile diabetes mellitus with proliferative diabetic retinopathy, and the other had bilateral retinal vasculitis of unknown etiology. Thus eight of ten patients in Group II (80%) investigated by carotid arteriography showed a severe carotid artery disease.

It is evident that in eyes with central retinal artery occlusion but no ocular neovascularization (Group I), at least half of the patients showed evidence of carotid artery disease on the same side. Embolism was probably responsible for their central retinal artery occlusion; the central retinal artery occlusion in the remaining patients of this group might have been due either to embolism (from the heart and, rarely, from hematologic disorders), spasm (from severe hypertension), or thrombosis of the central retinal artery. Thus embolism, particulary from the carotid arteries, is the most common cause of central retinal artery occlusion.

In nine patients from Group II, the central retinal artery occlusion was secondary to chronic ocular ischemia caused by severe carotid artery disease. As compared to the patients in Group I, these patients with chronic ocular ischemia showed some very distinctive features which include the following:

1. *Age*: These were much older patients; there were no young patients in this group.
2. *Mode of onset of visual loss*: This was usually either gradually progressive or preceded by recurrent attacks of amaurosis fugax instead of the dramatic sudden visual loss.
3. *Visual outcome*: Extremely poor.
4. *Carotid artery disease*: This was universally seen with complete occlusion or severe stenosis.
5. *Severe generalized atherosclerotic arterial disease*: Extremely common.

MECHANISM OF CENTRAL RETINAL ARTERY OCCLUSION IN CHRONIC OCULAR ISCHEMIA

In chronic ocular ischemia produced by occlusion or severe stenosis of the internal carotid artery, there is ischemia of both the anterior and posterior segments of the eye.

Anterior Segment Ischemia

It is well established that anterior segment ischemia causes neovascularization of the iris and angle, and this progresses to neovascular glaucoma. The rise of intraocular pressure varies considerably once neovascular glaucoma develops, and it is not uncommon to find no significant rise of intraocular pressure above "normal" levels because of the associated chronic ischemia of the ciliary body, thus leading one to believe that the eye does not have glaucoma.

Posterior Segment Ischemia

Internal carotid artery occlusion or severe stenosis, in the absence of adequate collateral circulation, must obviously produce an extreme fall in blood pressure in the central retinal artery and posterior ciliary arteries. The blood flow in the intraocular arteries depends on their perfusion pressure (perfusion pressure equals the mean blood pressure minus the intraocular pressure). Even if the intraocular pressure is "normal" or only moderately elevated, in the presence of a very low mean blood pressure in the central retinal artery, the circumstances are more than adequate to reduce the perfusion pressure to a low enough level to stop the retinal blood flow and produce central retinal artery occlusion. The subject is discussed at length elsewhere (1) and is represented diagrammatically in Figure 6.1.

DISCUSSION

In the past neovascular glaucoma was erroneously thought to be due to central retinal artery occlusion and the mechanism was considered to be identical to that of the neovascular glaucoma seen with central retinal vein occlusion. Our study (1) clearly demonstrated that this was not the case,

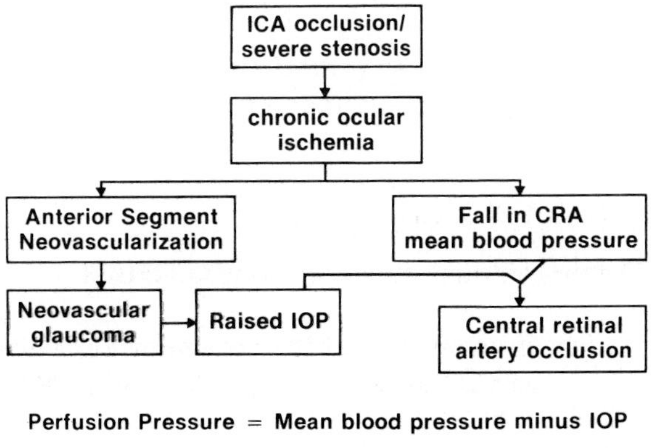

Fig. 6.1. Diagrammatic representation of sequence of events in eyes with central retinal artery (CRA) occlusion (CRAO), neovascular glaucoma (NVG), and carotid artery disease.

and that central retinal artery occlusion and neovascular glaucoma are not cause and effect. In fact, in the vast majority of patients, it is the neovascular glaucoma secondary to chronic ocular ischemia that caused central retinal artery occlusion.

Recently, Brown (2) disputed our conclusion on the basis of *one patient*, because on subtraction carotid angiography no carotid artery disease was detected and on fluorescein fundus angiography "normal choroidal filling" was seen. It is well established that a normal subtraction carotid angiogram and normal noninvasive tests do not rule out carotid artery disease, and also that filling of the choroid on fluorescein fundus angiography does not rule out ophthalmic artery insufficiency. Moreover, on rare occasions, chronic ocular ischemia can be produced by causes other than carotid artery disease or ophthalmic artery occlusion. Brown speculated that incomplete occlusion of the central retinal artery in his patient caused chronic retinal hypoxia and consequent ocular neovascularization; however, this speculation has no scientific basis because our clinical and experimental studies (3) on central retinal artery occlusion in a large volume of material have shown that the concept of "incomplete central retinal artery occlusion" is wrong. In view of these multiple problems with the case report by Brown, the conclusions drawn by the author are unwarranted and misleading.

Thus, all the evidence strongly points to carotid artery disease as the most frequent cause of iris and angle neovascularization, neovascular glaucoma, and associated central retinal artery occlusion, with central retinal artery occlusion usually being secondary to neovascular glaucoma and not vice versa.

Possibly, in some instances, an embolus from the diseased carotid arteries may produce central retinal artery occlusion, independent of the anterior segment ischemia and associated neovascularization, so that neovascular glaucoma and central retinal artery occlusion are two independent manifestations of carotid artery disease. The two may develop almost simultaneously or central retinal artery occlusion may precede the development of neovascularization of the anterior segment and neovascular glaucoma. This is further suggested by the fact that sometimes the interval between the central retinal artery occlusion and development of neovascular glaucoma may be about a year or longer.

CONCLUSIONS

From our studies it can be concluded that:

(a) In two-thirds of the patients with central retinal artery occlusion, carotid artery disease was responsible for the occlusion.

(b) Central retinal artery occlusion or neovascular glaucoma may be the earliest clinical signs of serious carotid artery disease, requiring urgent carotid artery evaluation by reliable techniques.
(c) Absence of any abnormality on noninvasive tests for carotid artery disease *does not rule out carotid artery disease*, as these tests are totally unreliable and of little value in investigation of central retinal artery occlusion.

ACKNOWLEDGMENT

I am grateful to Mrs. Georgiane Parkes-Perret for the secretarial help.

This investigation was supported by grant EY-01151 from the National Institutes of Health, Bethesda, MD.

REFERENCES

1. Hayreh, S.S., and Podhajsky, P.: Ocular neovascularization with retinal vascular occlusion. II. Occurrence in central and branch retinal artery occlusion. *Arch. Ophthalmol.* 100:1585, 1982.
2. Brown, G.C.: Isolated central retinal artery obstruction in association with ocular neovascularization. *Am. J. Ophthalmol.* 96:110, 1983.
3. Hayreh, S.S., and Weingeist, T.A.: Experimental occlusion of the central artery of the retina. I. Ophthalmoscopic and fluorescein fundus angiographic studies. *Br. J. Ophthalmol.* 64:896, 1980.

7

FLUORESCEIN ANGIOGRAPHY IN OCULAR ISCHEMIA SYNDROMES

Harold Weiss, M.D., F.A.C.S.
Reed M. Bouchey, B.S.*

Fluorescein angiography was described in 1961 by Novotny and Alvis (1) as a technique for visualizing the retinal vasculature. Soon thereafter, Hollenhorst and Kearns (2), David (3), and Pemberton (4) described using sodium fluorescein for measuring arm-to-retina circulation time in patients with carotid occlusive disease.

In 1966, David et al. elaborated on the use of intravenous fluorescein for evaluating carotid occlusive disease. They emphasized not only the importance of the arm-to-retina circulation time and the first appearance of the dye in the retinal arteries, but also careful observation of the fluorescein transit through the entire retinal circulation, especially watching the venous filling phase. By following the venous phase of the angiogram, David found it was much easier to identify ocular hypoperfusion than by watching for the critical moment when fluorescein dye first appeared in the retinal vessels. He tested a series of normal patients and found an arm-to-retina circulation time of about 11 seconds. The onset of early venous filling appeared at 13 seconds, and the onset of late venous phase appeared at about 18 seconds. He then observed the fluorescein angiographic timing in normal patients in whom digital compression to the carotid artery was applied. Digital compression delayed *all* phases of the angiogram. He also evaluated two patients with carotid artery occlusion which had been confirmed by angiography. He found essentially the same pattern of delayed onset of both the arterial and venous phases.

In 1968 Newsome et al. experimentally created carotid artery occlusions in rhesus monkeys. They then watched the pattern of the fluorescein angiogram with particular emphasis on the venous phase of the angiogram.

*School of Medicine, Wayne State University, Detroit, Michigan

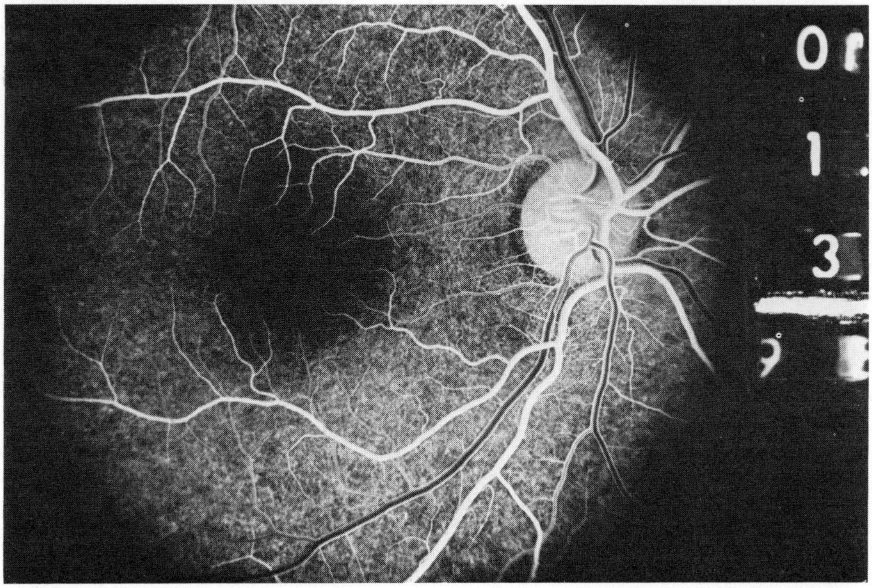

Fig. 7.1. Early fluorescein angiogram at 12.3 seconds showing contrast medium filling the major retinal arterioles and some of the branch arterioles. There is some very early laminar flow in the veins.

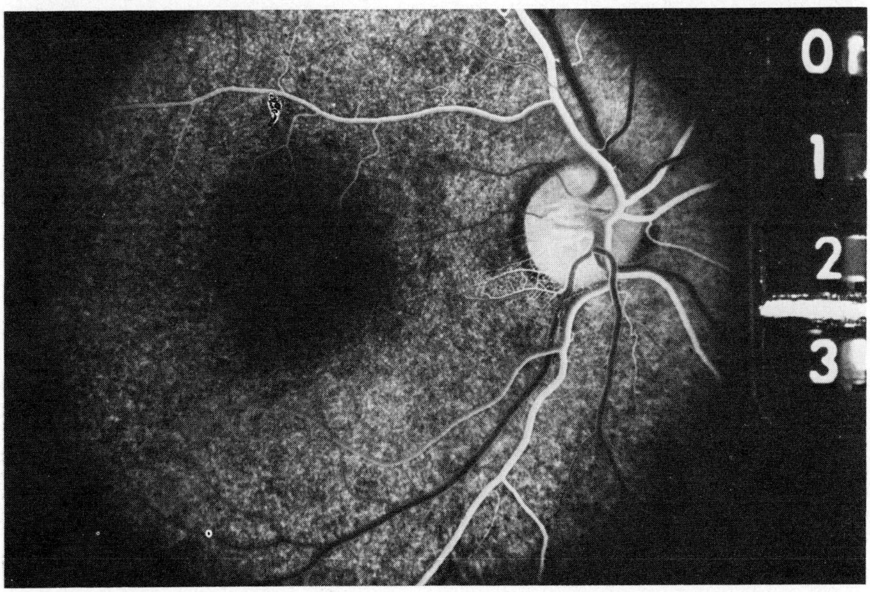

Fig. 7.2. Early venous phase at 13.9 seconds with more filling of the small arterioles, venules and prominent laminar flow in the major veins.

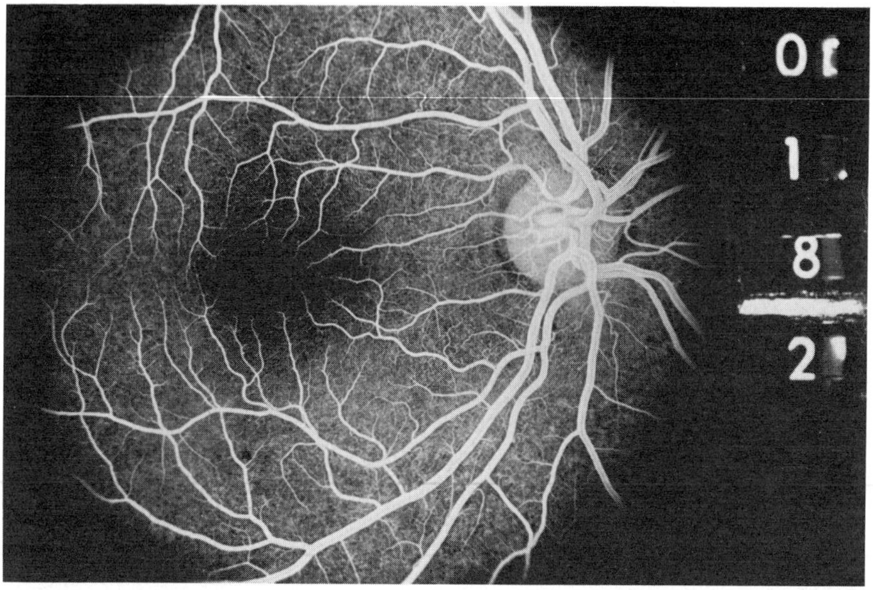

Fig. 7.3. Mid-venous phase at 18.2 seconds showing prominent filling of the entire retinal capillary bed and contrast medium filling the major veins almost completely.

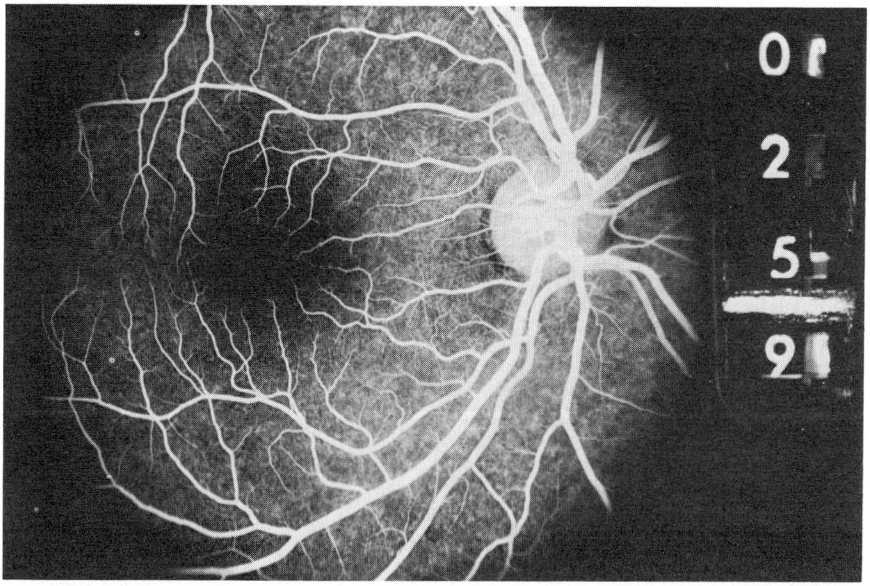

Fig. 7.4. By 25.9 seconds, fluorescein dye completely fills the major veins.

His findings were similar to those of David: a prolongation of the development of all the phases of the angiogram, venous as well as arterial.

However, clinical experience with fluorescein angiography over the years has shown that the test is of less value in the diagnosis of carotid artery disease than such tests as ophthalmodynamometry, oculoplethysmography, phonoangiography and real-time ultrasonography. Fluorescein angiography fell out of favor as a test for the primary evaluation of extraocular vascular disease.

The purpose of this paper is not to resurrect fluorescein angiography as a test for the evaluation of carotid artery disease, but rather to heighten awareness among ophthalmologists that the fluorescein angiogram may reflect extraocular vascular disease and that the timing of fluorescein transit through the retinal circulation should always be given attention.

A brief review of the normal sequence and timing of a fluorescein angiogram is shown in Figures 7.1 to 7.4.

We will present a series of patients who came to Retina Service of the Kresge Eye Institute with ocular symptoms which proved to be due to extraocular vascular disease. The purpose of these presentations is to show that ophthalmologists must maintain a ready awareness of the impact of vascular supply to the eye in evaluating ocular disease.

CASE REPORTS

Case 1

A 52-year-old white woman was referred to our service with decreased vision in the right eye of three days duration, due to "macular edema." The patient had had an intracapsular cataract extraction in the right eye one month prior. There was no other significant medical or surgical history.

Visual acuity was finger counting O.D. and 20/25 O.S. The anterior segment was unremarkable except for aphakia. Fundus examination demonstrated mild whitening of the macular area (Figure 7.5). Fluorescein angiography demonstrated a marked delay in onset of arterial perfusion as well as a marked decrease in intraretinal transit time (Figures 7.6 to 7.9). Four-vessel arteriography showed a normal carotid bifurcation (Figure 7.10). Magnification views of the orbit, however, demonstrated marked irregularity of the ophthalmic artery (Figure 7.11). The patient was treated with persantine and aspirin. Three weeks later, her vision had improved to 20/60 O.D. On fundus examination, the macular whitening had resolved. Two months later, her ocular status was unchanged.

The patient's presumptive diagnosis on referral was "macular edema."

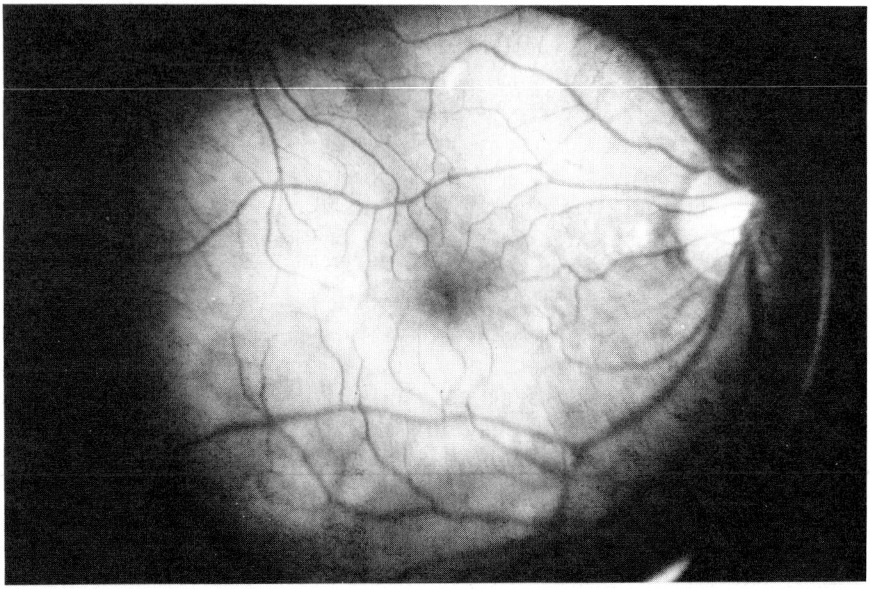

Fig. 7.5. Fundus photograph of the right eye showing edema of the retina and the posterior pole.

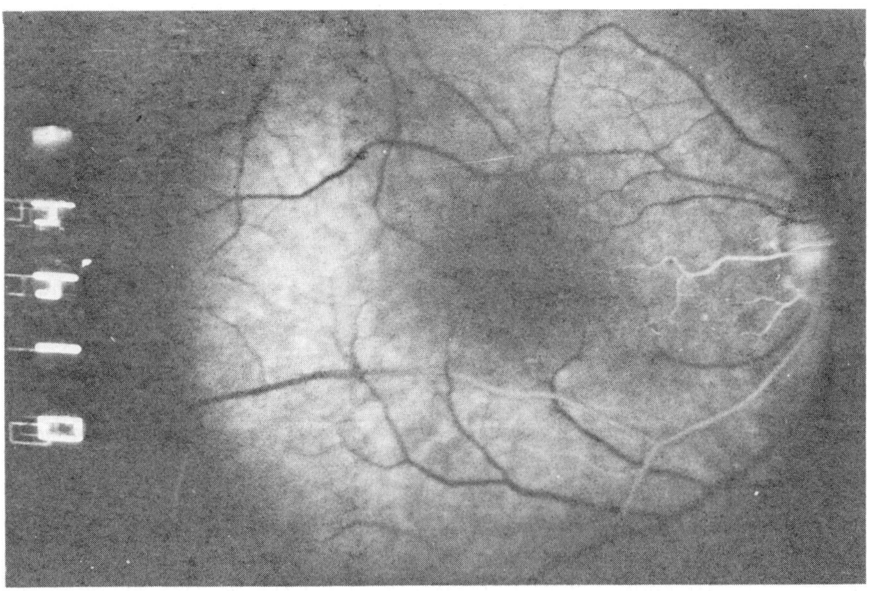

Fig. 7.6. Early fluorescein angiogram at 14.4 seconds shows background choroidal filling but very slow filling of the major arterioles.

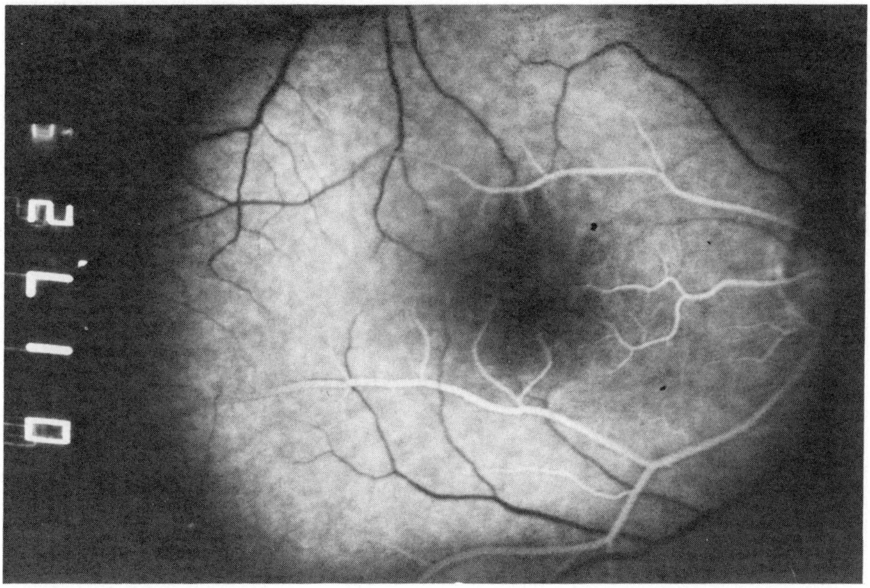

Fig. 7.7. Three seconds later, there is still only early arterial filling. Normally, by this stage, there would already be filling in the major veins as well.

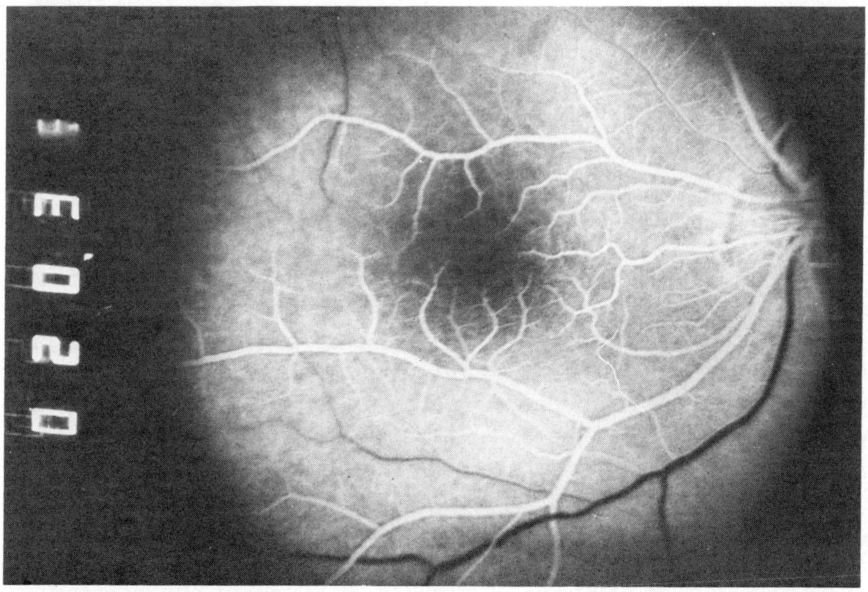

Fig. 7.8. At 0.3 seconds, approximately 6 seconds after the onset of early arterial filling, we are still barely into the venous phase of the angiogram. Normally, this picture would be seen 2–3 seconds after the onset of early arterial filling.

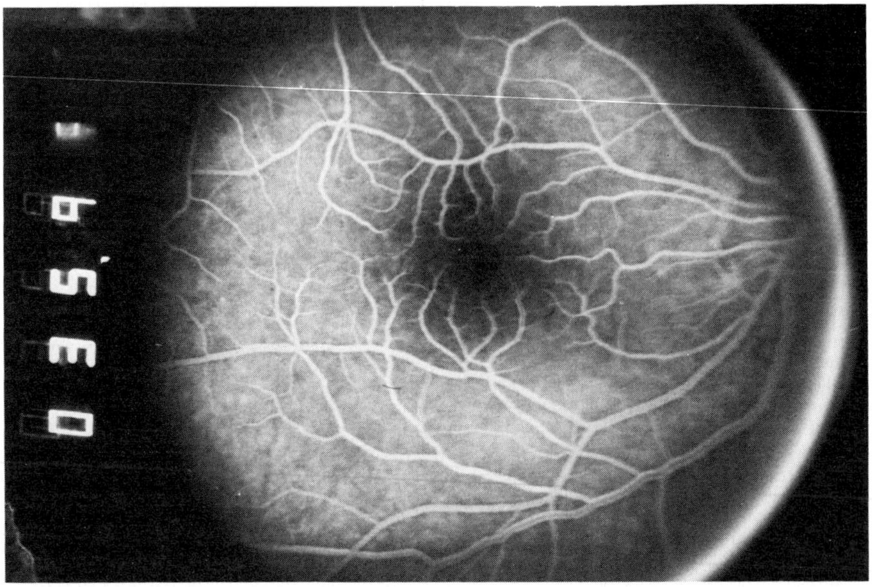

Fig. 7.9. By 35.9 seconds, we are still on the intermediate venous phase with laminar flow still visible in the major inferotemporal vein. Normally, by this stage, the veins should be completely filled with fluorescein (compare to Figure 7.4).

However, what was found on fluorescein angiography was the ocular equivalent of preinfarction angina. This observation led to prompt arteriography. Although a surgical lesion was not found, medical treatment may have been beneficial in preserving this patient's vision.

Case II

A 67-year-old white man presented with a two day history of intermittent blurring of vision in the right eye. He had had no previous significant history of ocular disease. On initial examination, vision fluctuated dramatically between 20/40 and 20/400. Anterior segment examination was normal. On fundus examination, there was prominent whitening of the retina in a patchy pattern in the posterior pole (Figure 7.12). We observed considerable sludging of blood flow through the retinal arterioles and venules. Fluorescein angiography demonstrated marked delay in the arterial and venous phases of the angiogram (Figures 7.13, 7.14). It was felt that this was a potentially salvageable partial central retinal artery obstruction. The patient was immediately hospitalized and heparinized. He underwent four-vessel arteriography which demonstrated a small

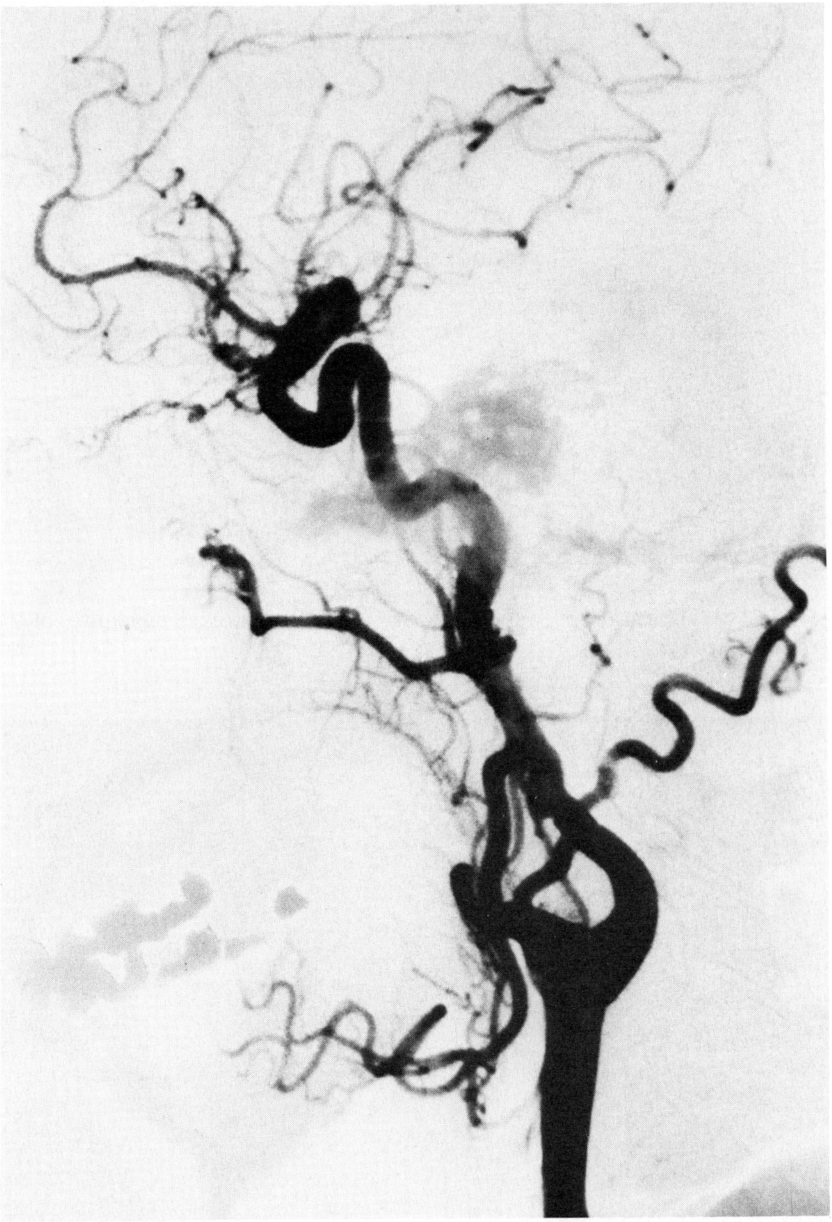

Fig. 7.10. Carotid arteriogram showing a relatively normal carotid bifurcation.

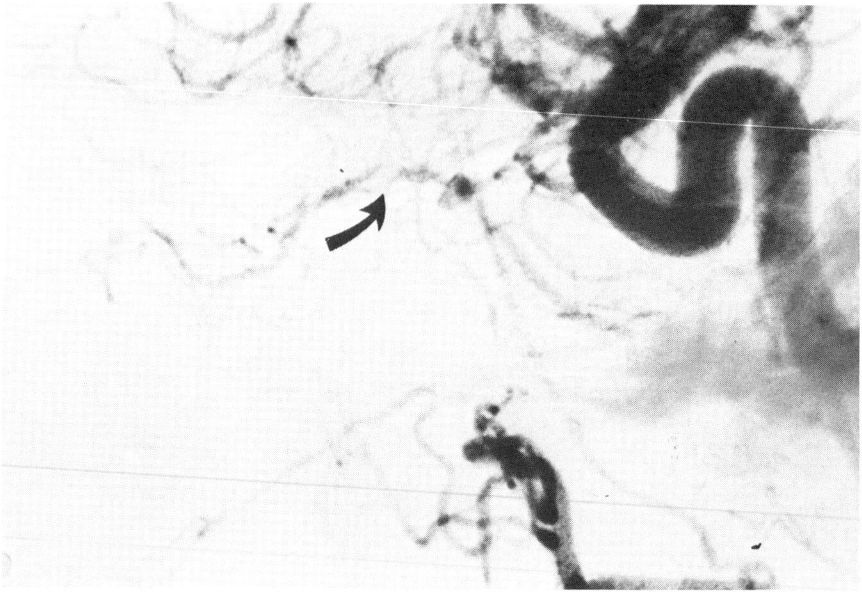

Fig. 7.11. Magnification views of the orbit show marked irregularity of the ophthalmic artery.

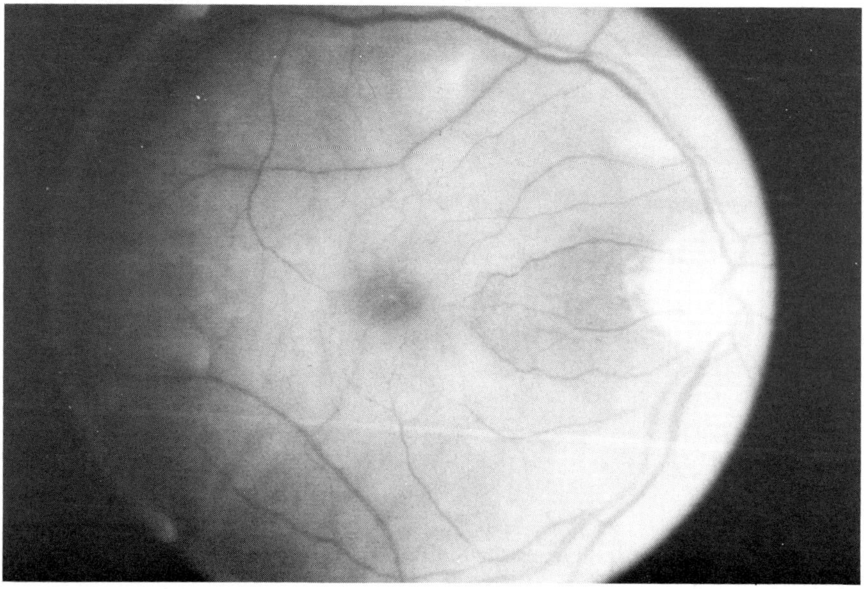

Fig. 7.12. Fundus photograph of the right eye showing patchy edema and whitening of the posterior pole.

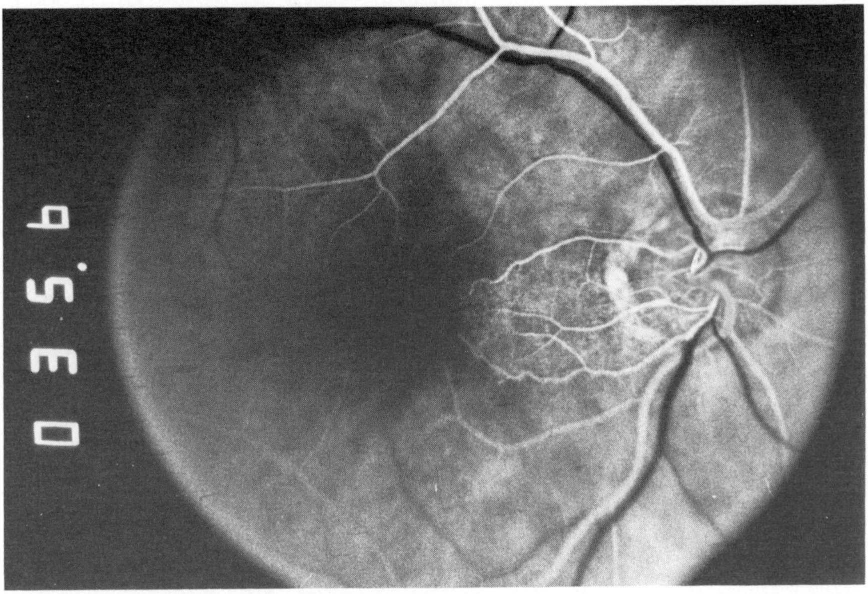

Fig. 7.13. At 35.6 seconds into the arteriogram, only the early arterial phase is seen. Normally, this phase of the angiogram would be seen at 12 to 14 seconds.

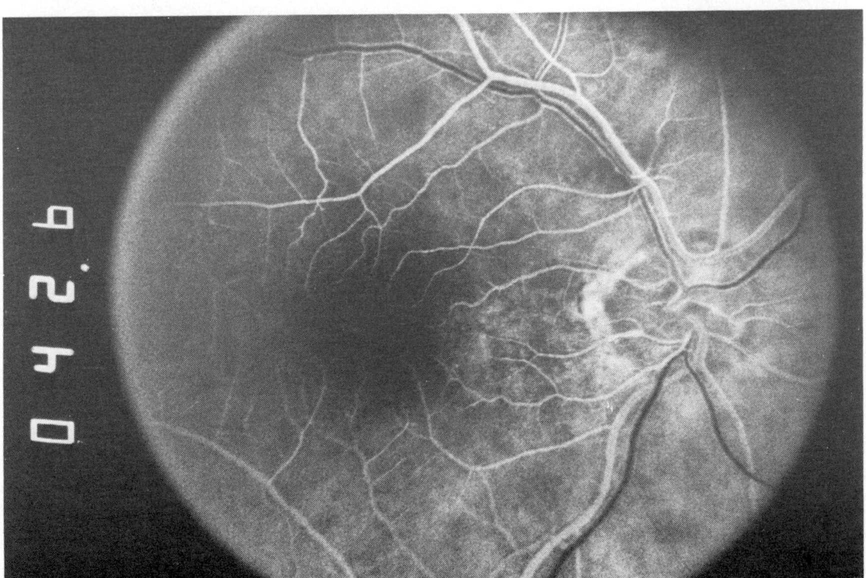

Fig. 7.14. Early laminar filling is still very prominent at 42.6 seconds demonstrating a marked delay in intraretinal transit time.

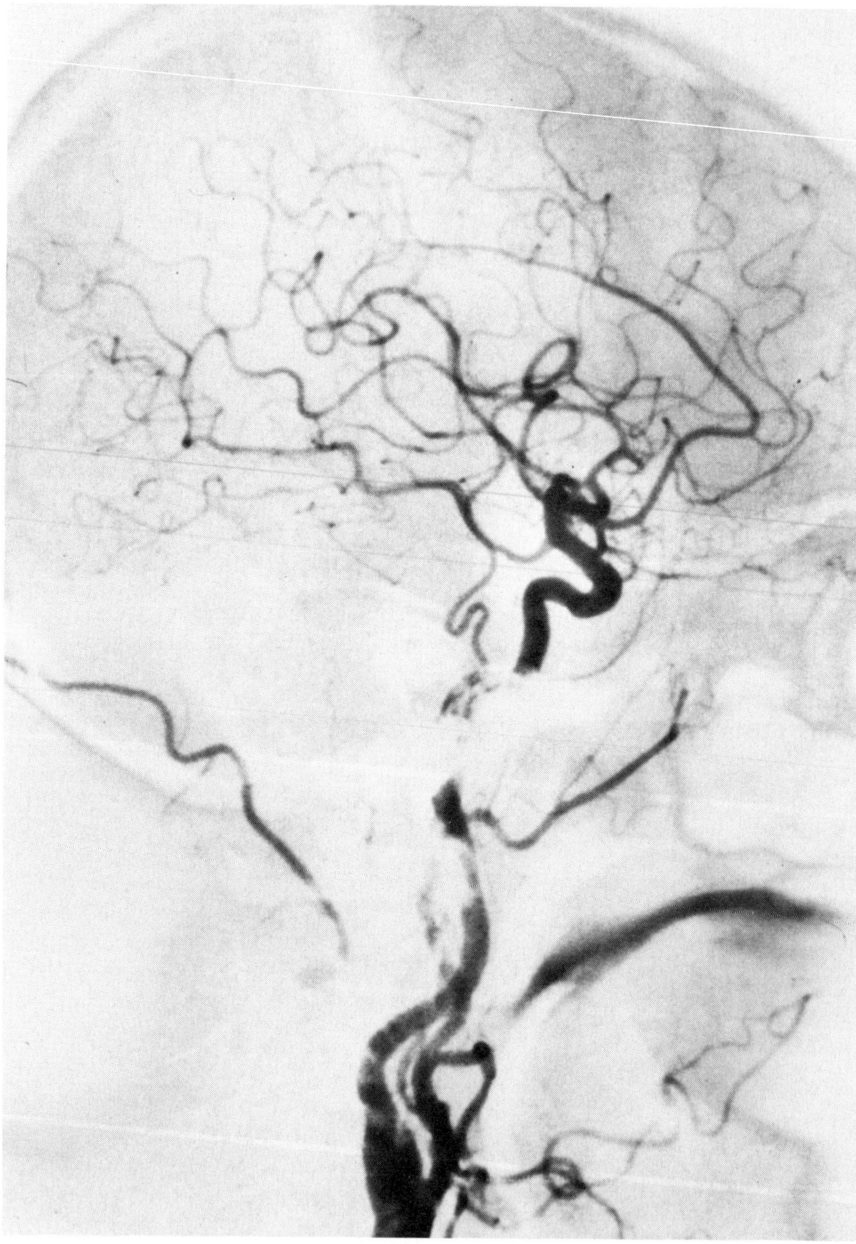

Fig. 7.15. Carotid arteriogram demonstrates subtle irregularities in the internal carotid artery.

plaque in the internal carotid artery (Figure 7.15.) The patient was taken immediately to the operating room, where a carotid endarterectomy was performed. At the time of surgery, a 2-cm ulcerated plaque was discovered and successfully removed. Two months post-operatively, the patient was doing well. Vision in the right eye had improved to 20/60 and has remained stable since that time.

This patient demonstrated an impending central retinal artery occlusion which was probably embolic in nature. Fluorescein angiography was helpful in showing that a reasonable amount of perfusion remained in the central retinal artery, and that aggressive treatment was indicated.

Case III

A 77-year-old white woman presented with loss of the lower half of the vision in her left eye of three hours duration. Vision was measured at 20/30 O.D. and 20/400 O.S. On fundus examination, there was a soft embolus present in the branches of the superior retinal artery and moderate whitening of the superior half of the retina (Figure 7.16). Fluorescein angiography demonstrated extremely delayed arterial perfusion with dye visible only after about 24 seconds. There was also a delay in the evolution of the venous phase. A filling defect was visible in the superior temporal and superior nasal arteries, outlining the embolus (Figures 7.17–7.19). The patient was admitted to the hospital and underwent four-vessel arteriography, which revealed total occlusion of the left internal carotid artery (Figure 7.20). Collateral flow was found to be supplying the cerebral and ophthalmic circulation on the left side.

Fluorescein angiography in this case was useful in showing not only evidence of embolism, but also of marked delay in perfusion, suggesting not only embolism, but also hemodynamically significant vascular obstruction.

Case IV

A 57-year-old white women presented with a four week history of decreasing vision in the left eye and "macular edema." The patient had a history of chronic, open-angle glaucoma which was being treated with Timoptic 0.5%.

On ocular examination, the patient's vision was 20/20 O.D. and finger counting O.S. There was a positive afferent conduction defect on the left. The anterior segment was normal. On fundus examination, there was evidence of a cilio-retinal artery occlusion, and of significant "venous stasis" with darkening and dilation of the retinal veins and punctate intraretinal hemorrhages throughout the fundus (Figure 7.21). Fluorescein angiography demonstrated a marked delay in the onset of retinal arterial

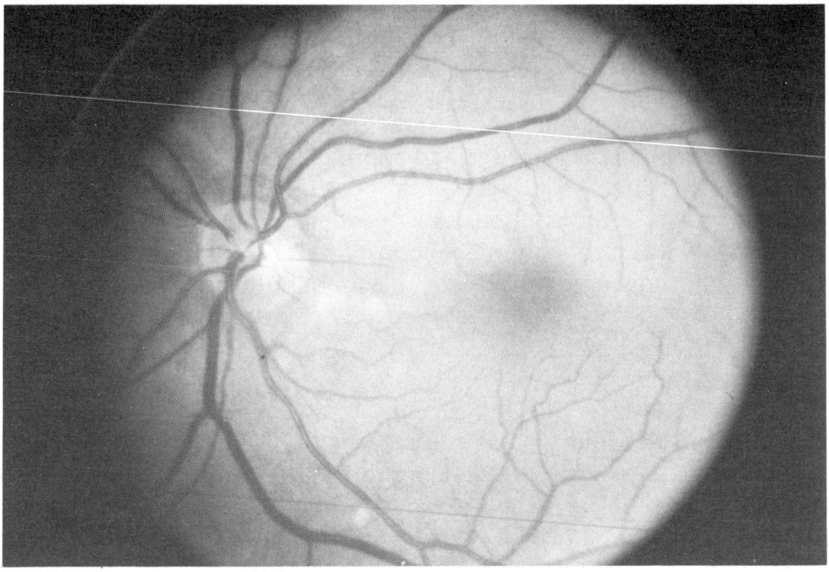

Fig. 7.16. Fundus photograph of the left eye showing a soft grey-white embolus present in the central retinal artery overlying the disc.

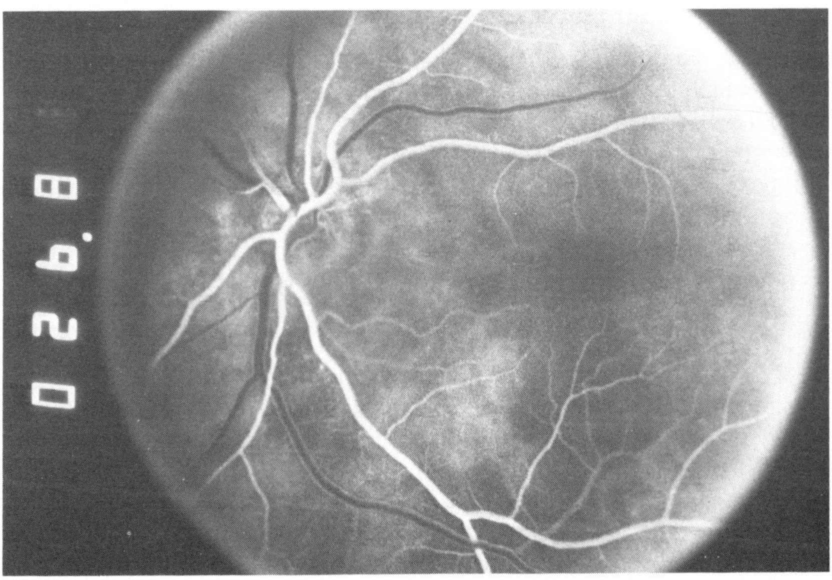

Fig. 7.17. Early fluorescein angiogram showing the filling defect from the embolus, especially prominent in the superior branches of the central retinal artery. Delayed filling of the superonasal arteriole is especially prominent. In addition to the visible embolus, the fact that the angiogram is only at the early venous phase at 26.8 seconds also strongly suggests a generalized perfusion defect to the eye.

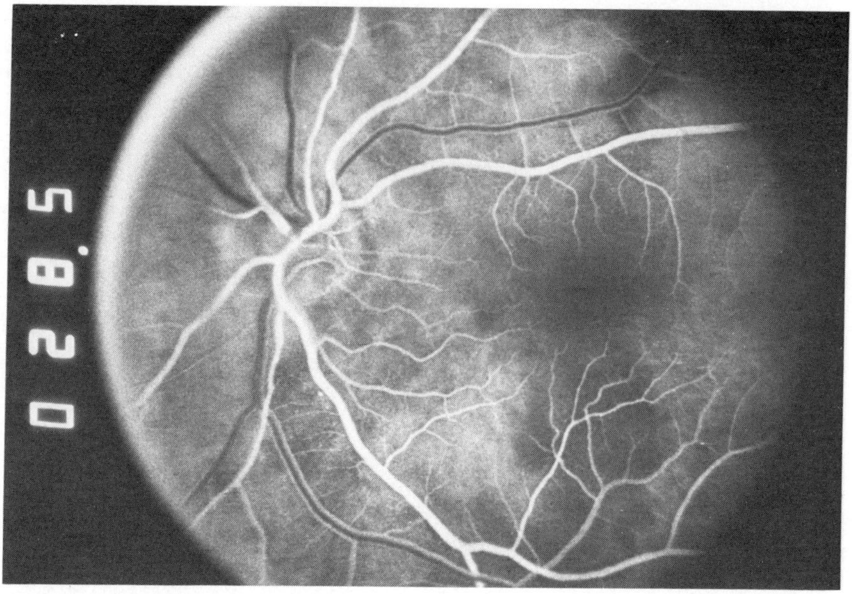

Fig. 7.18. At 28.5 seconds, there is still delayed venous return as well as relative hypofluorescence of the choroid, suggesting delayed choroidal filling as well as delayed central retinal artery filling.

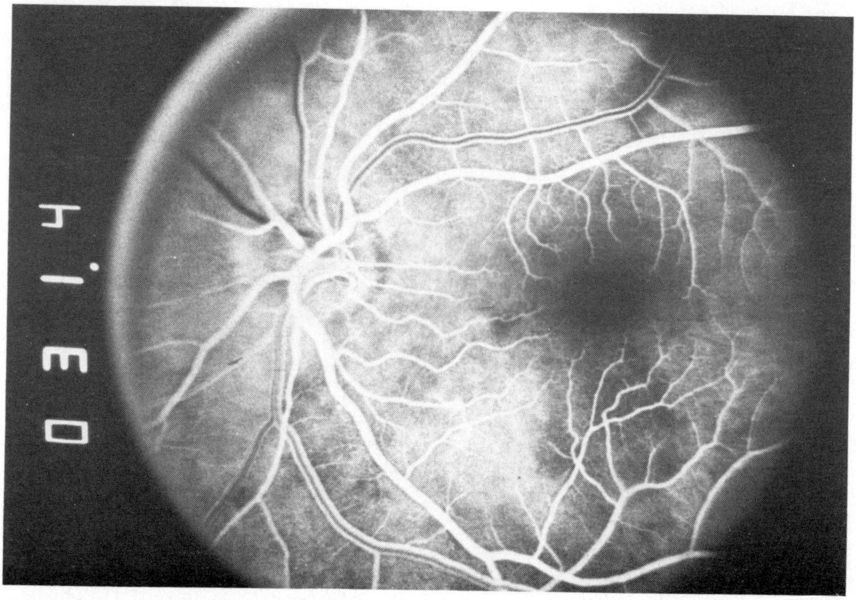

Fig. 7.19. Choroidal filling and retinal capillary filling are both improving but at a much later time than is normal.

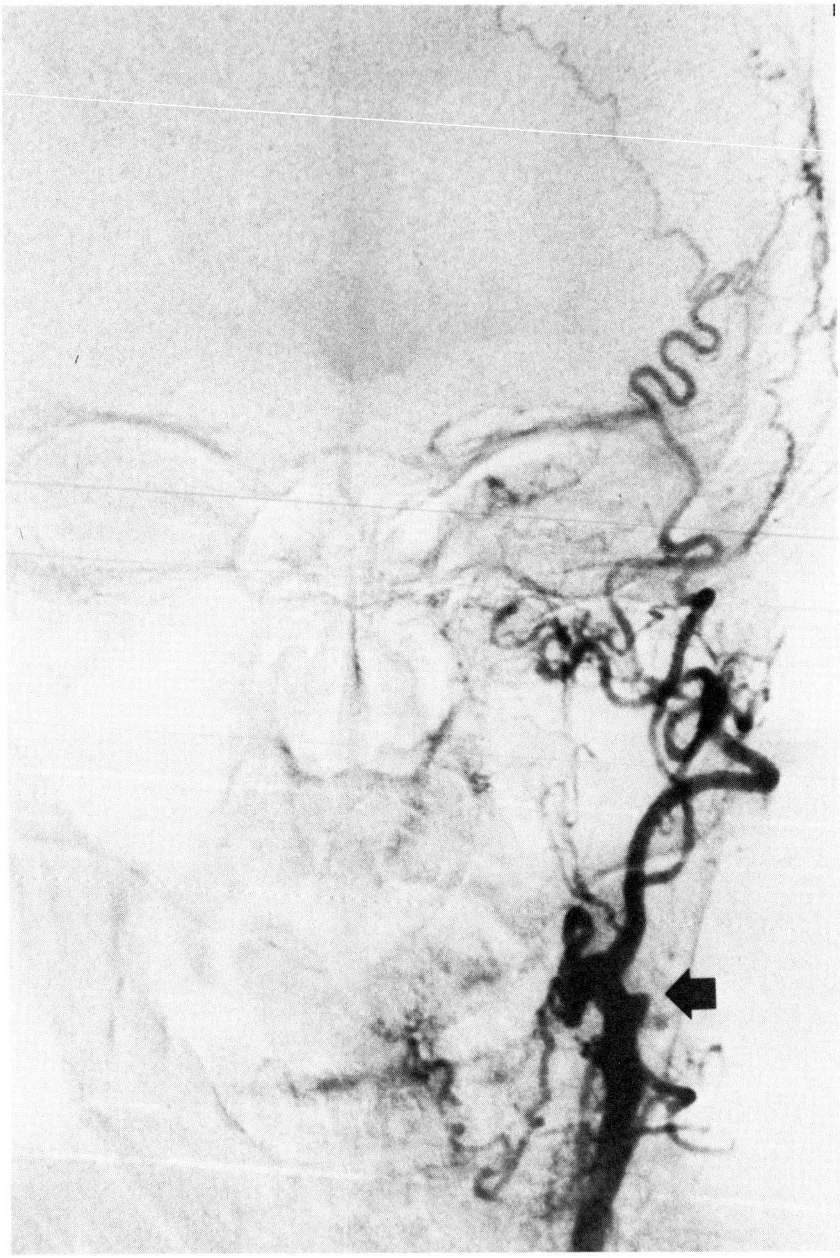

Fig. 7.20. Arteriography demonstrates a total occlusion of the left internal carotid artery (arrow).

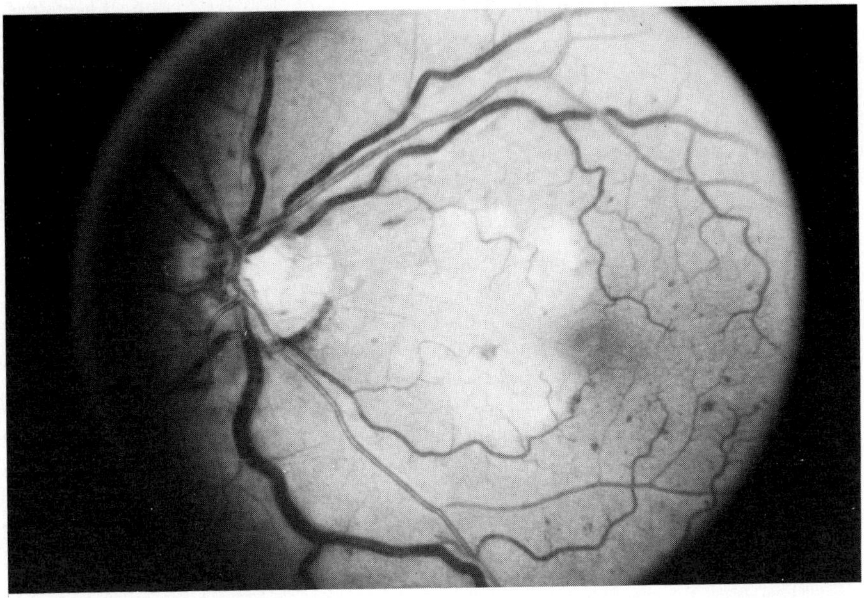

Fig. 7.21. Fundus photograph of the left eye showing whitening of the retina in the papillo-macular bundle and also evidence of venous statis with darkening and dilation of the venous system and punctate hemorrhages throughout the retina.

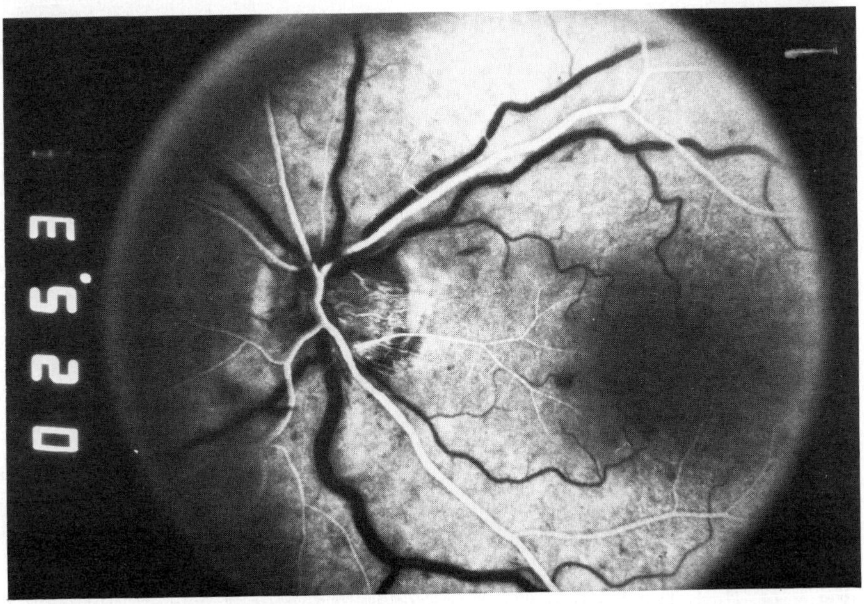

Fig. 7.22. Fluorescein angiogram at 25.3 seconds is still in the arterial phase with no venous filling yet visible. This is a delay of approximately two times normal in the onset of early arterial filling.

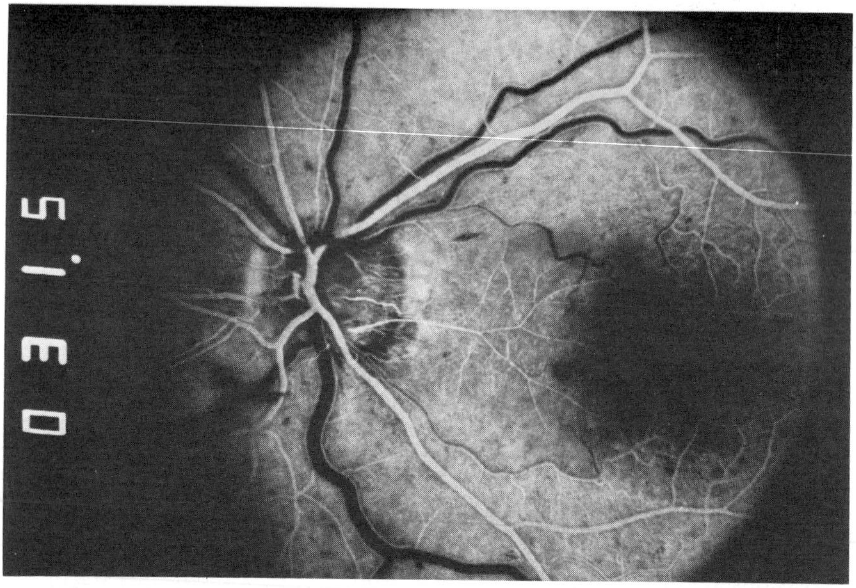

Fig. 7.23. At 31.5 seconds, only very early venous filling is seen. Normally, this would be seen 1 to 2 seconds after the arterial phase begins. Flow through the small cilioretinal vessel is extremely irregular.

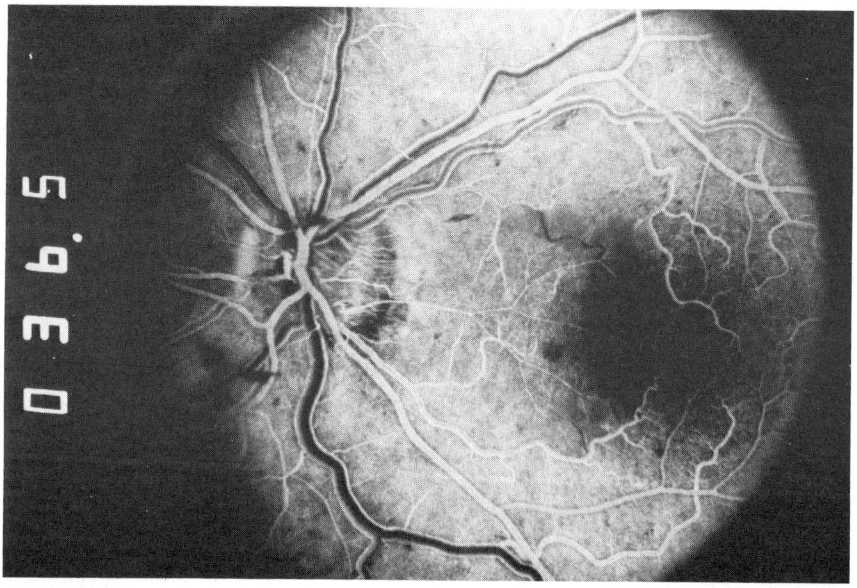

Fig. 7.24. Early laminar flow is still present at 36.5 seconds, whereas normally, the veins would be completely filled with dye. Prominent delayed flow through the obstructed segment of retina, supplied by the cilioretinal artery, is quite prominent.

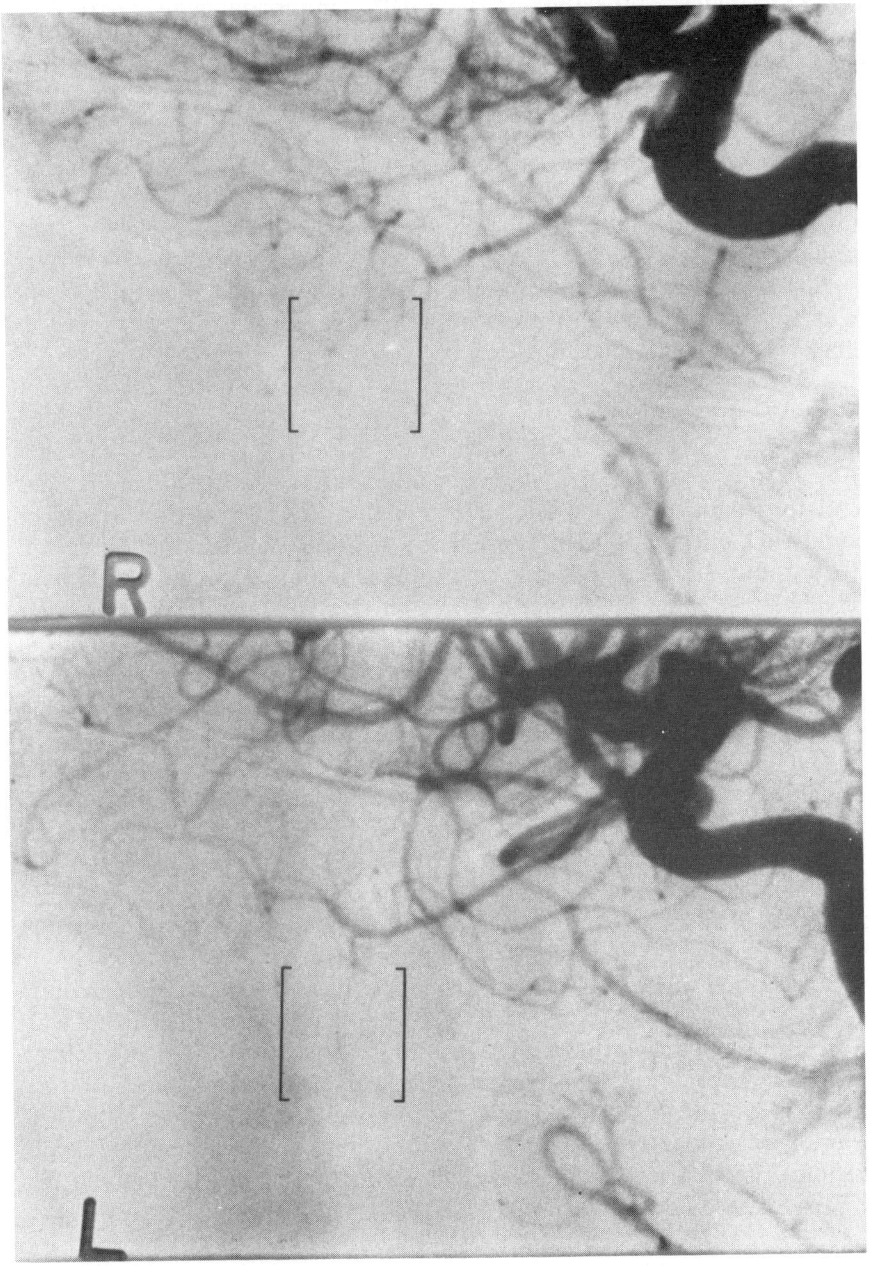

Fig. 7.25. Orbital subtraction films comparing the right and left eyes show a relative absence of ciliary vessels on the left side compared to the right side (compare the area between brackets).

and venous phases of the angiogram as well as moderate delay in choroidal filling. The involved cilioretinal artery was extremely thin and irregular (Figures 7.22–7.24). Four-vessel arteriography was performed, which showed no abnormalities of the common carotid artery or the carotid bifurcation. Careful evaluation of the orbital subtraction films was interpreted as showing an absence of the posterior ciliary vessels on the left side compared to the right side (Figure 7.25). The patient was treated conservatively with platelet inhibitors. Her central vision in the left eye has remained reduced.

Fluorescein angiogram showed evidence of not only cilioretinal artery occlusion, but also significant obstruction in the central retinal artery as well as the posterior ciliary arteries.

Case V

A 79-year-old white man had intermittent blurring of vision in the right eye of four days duration. Ocular examination revealed a visual cuity of 20/100 O.D. and 20/50 O.S. There was a right afferent conduction defect. Slit lamp examination was unremarkable. Fundus examination demonstrated pale swelling of the optic disc with peripapillary nerve fiber layer hemorrhages (Figure 7.26). Fluorescein angiography demonstrated dilation of some of the epipapillary capillaries, loss of perfusion in other aspects of the optic disc and extensive late leakage (Figures 7.27–7.29). There was no apparent delay in central retinal arterial perfusion.

The patient underwent four-vessel arteriography, which demonstrated an ulcerated plaque with stenosis near the origin of the right internal carotid artery (Figure 7.30). Subtraction films of the orbit demonstrated loss of the posterior ciliary branches of the right ophthalmic artery (Figure 7.31). The patient underwent right internal carotid endarterectomy and recovered uneventfully from surgery. His vision has remained stable in the right eye. He has developed no symptoms in his opposite eye.

This patient raises the issue of the association between ischemic optic neuropathy and carotid vascular disease. A subpopulation of patients with ischemic optic neuropathy may have embolization to the posterior ciliary vessels as a cause of acute ischemic optic neuropathy. Also carotid artery disease may further compromise existing small vessel disease of the posterior ciliary vessels and thereby contribute to or precipitate acute ischemic optic neuropathy. This issue has been discussed elsewhere in this symposium, and certainly warrants further investigation.

Case VI

A 57-year-old white woman with a 15 year history of diabetes mellitus was referred for floaters in her left eye of one month duration. Patient had a

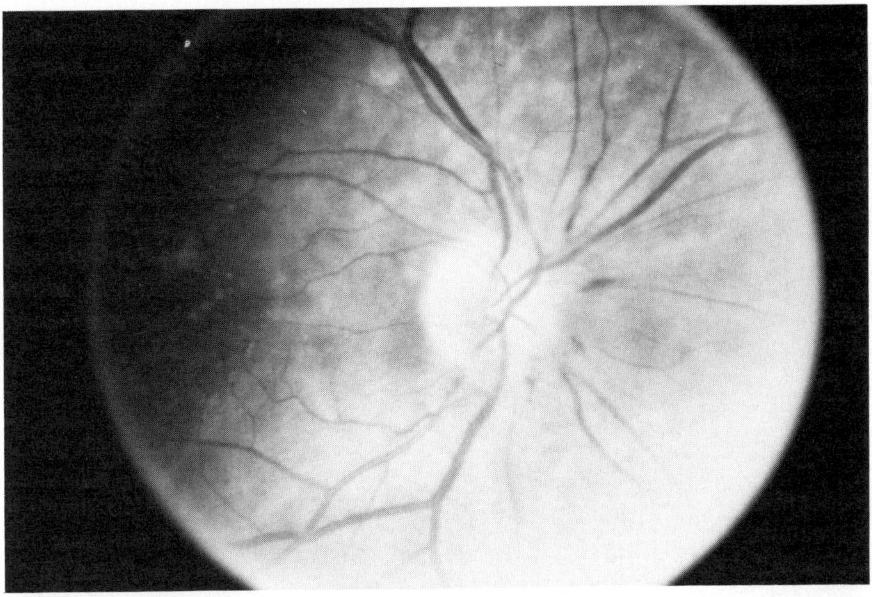

Fig. 7.26. Fundus photograph of the right eye shows mild optic disc swelling with peripapillary nerve fiber layer hemorrhages.

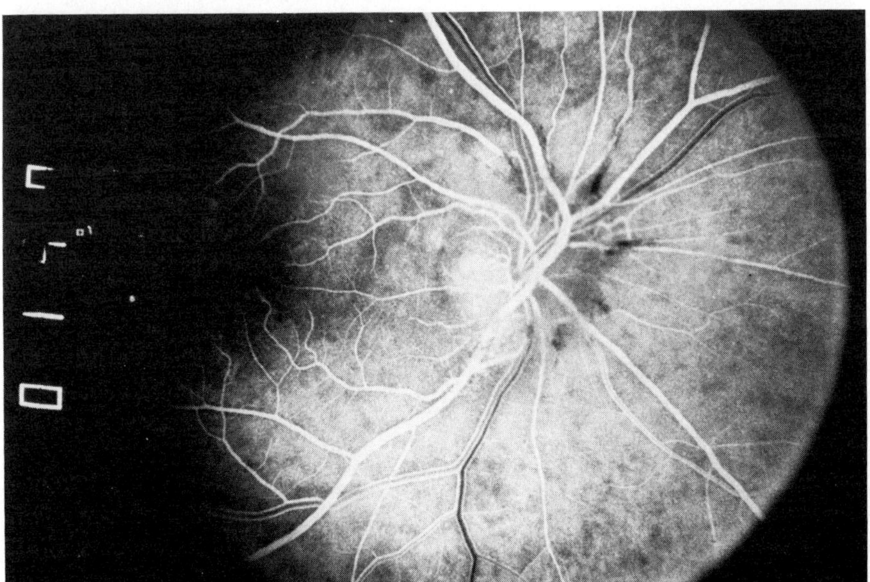

Fig. 7.27. Early angiogram shows dilation of the epipapillary capillaries from the 6 to 9 o'clock area on the disc and relative hypoperfusion of the capillaries on the nasal side of the disc.

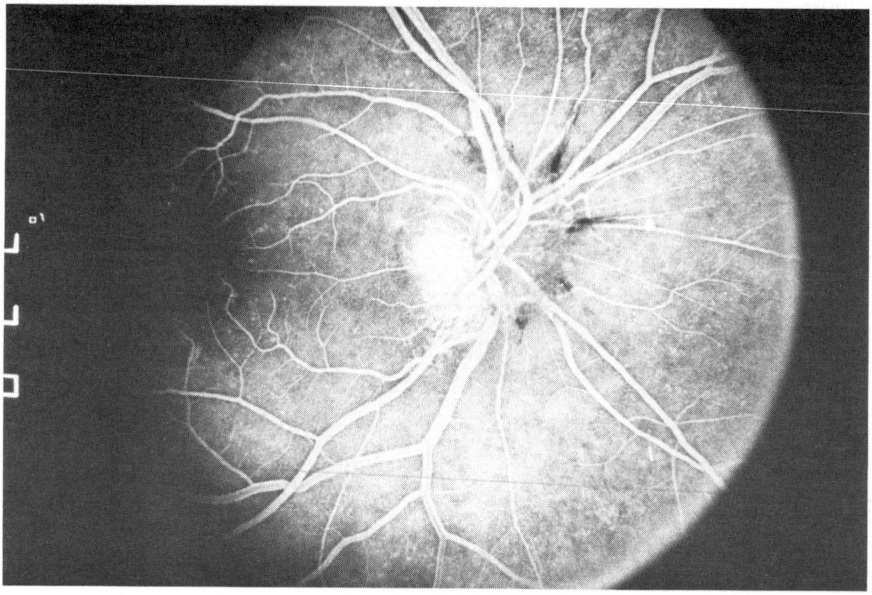

Fig. 7.28. Delayed perfusion to the nasal side of the disc continues.

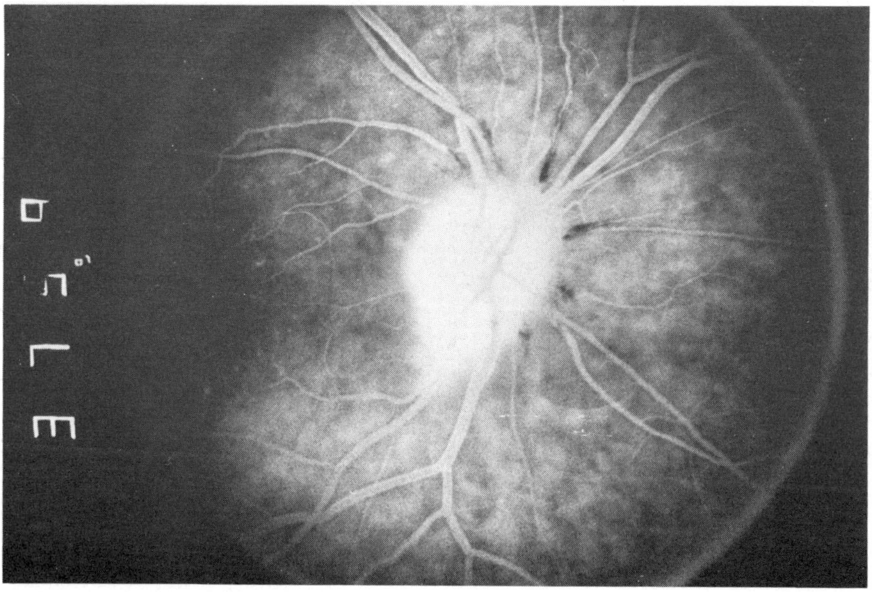

Fig. 7.29. Late angiogram showing extensive leakage of fluorescein and "staining" of the disc with fluorescein.

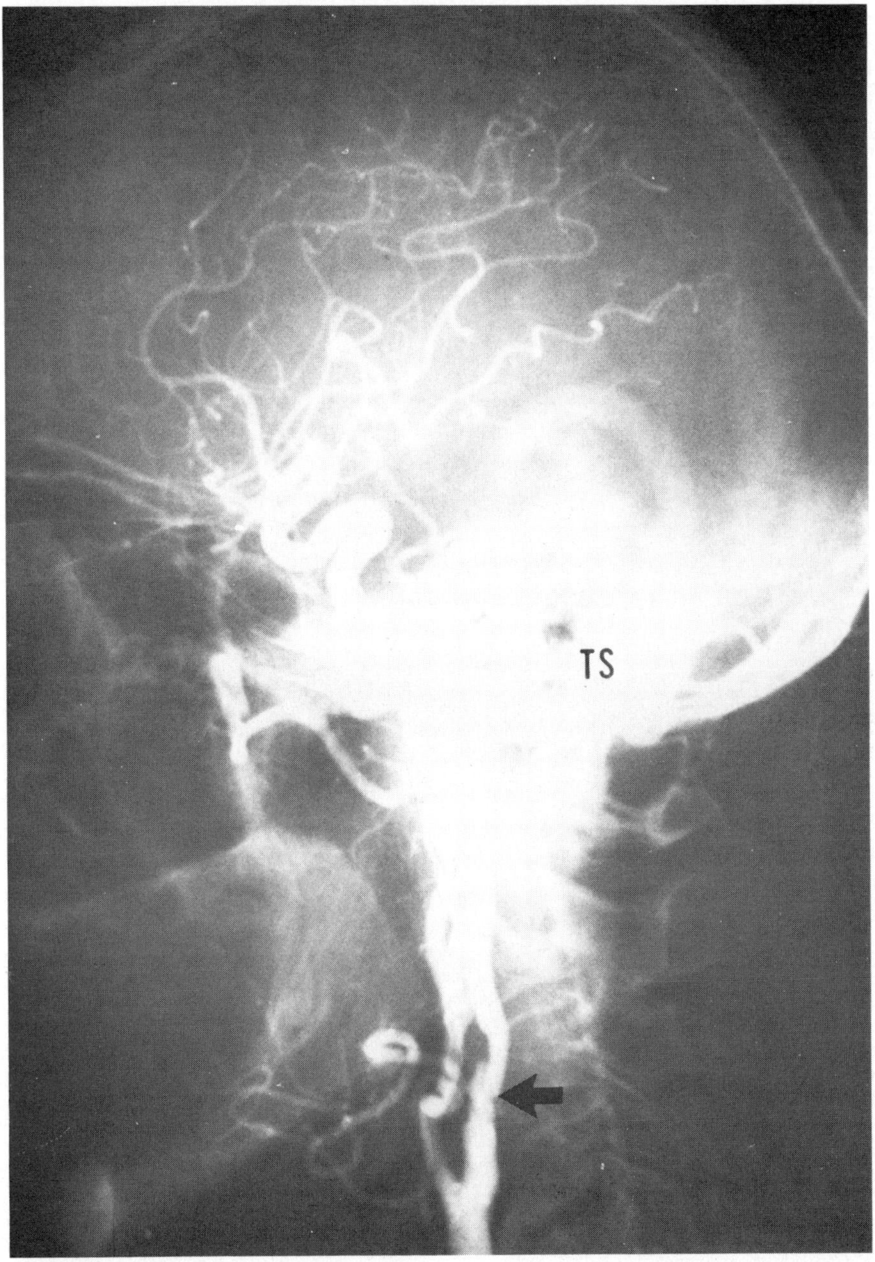

Fig. 7.30. Arteriography demonstrates an ulcerated plaque with stenosis near the origin of the right internal carotid artery (*arrow*).

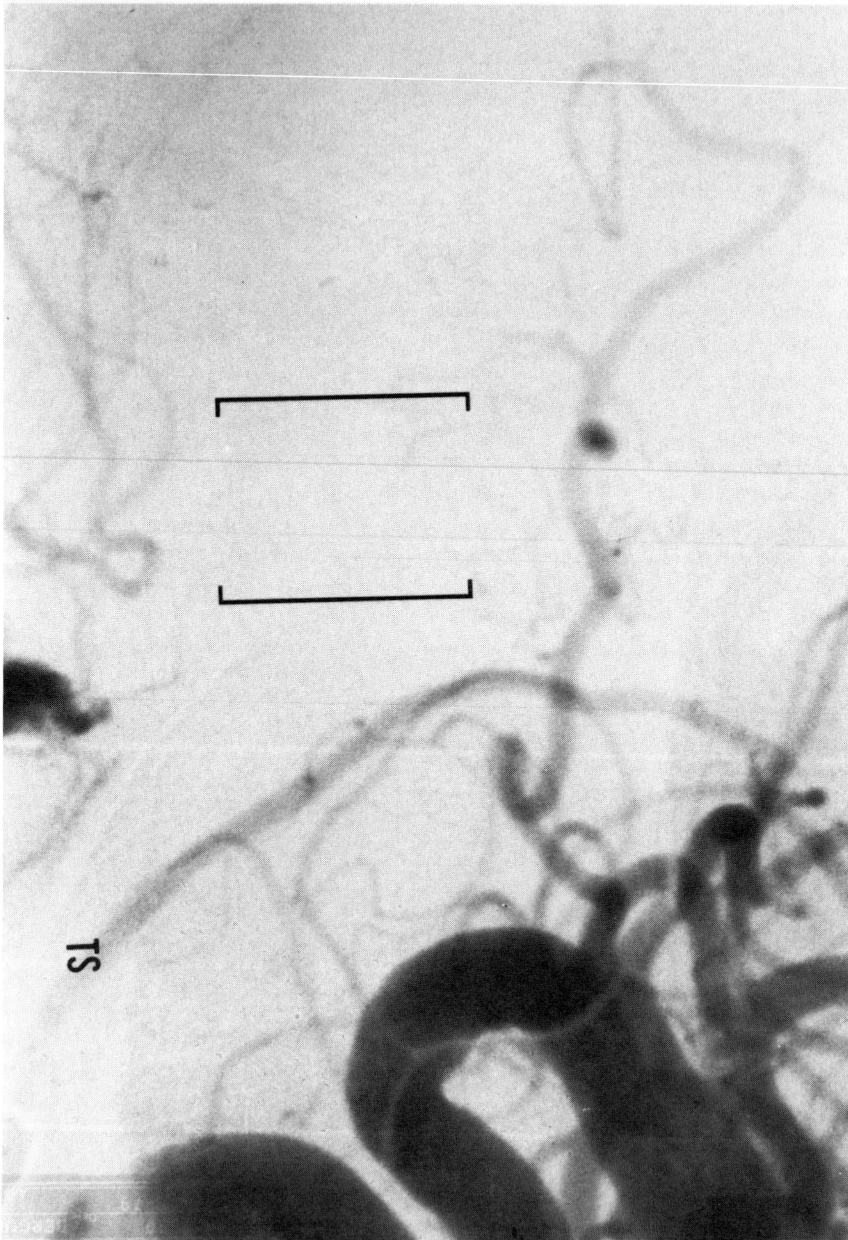

Fig. 7.31. Subtraction films of the orbit demonstrate a relative loss of posterior ciliary vessels in the right orbit (area between brackets).

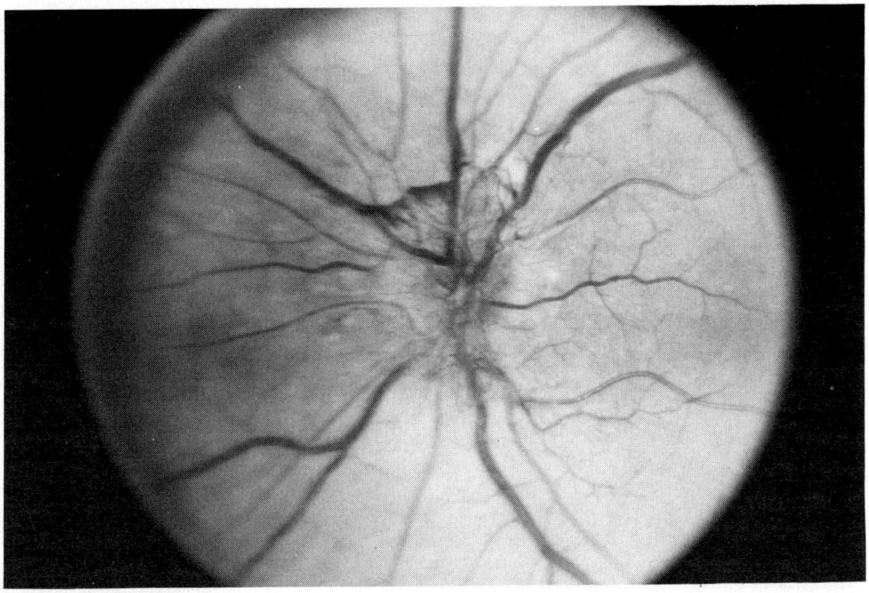

Fig. 7.32. Fundus photograph of the left eye showing extensive optic disc neovascularization.

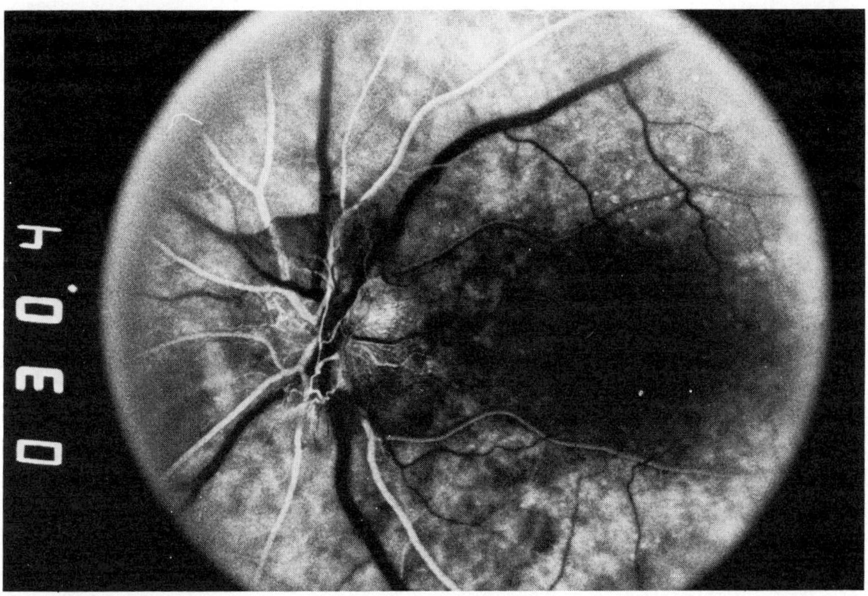

Fig. 7.33. Early fluorescein angiogram shows early arterial filling at 30.4 seconds, which is a marked delay.

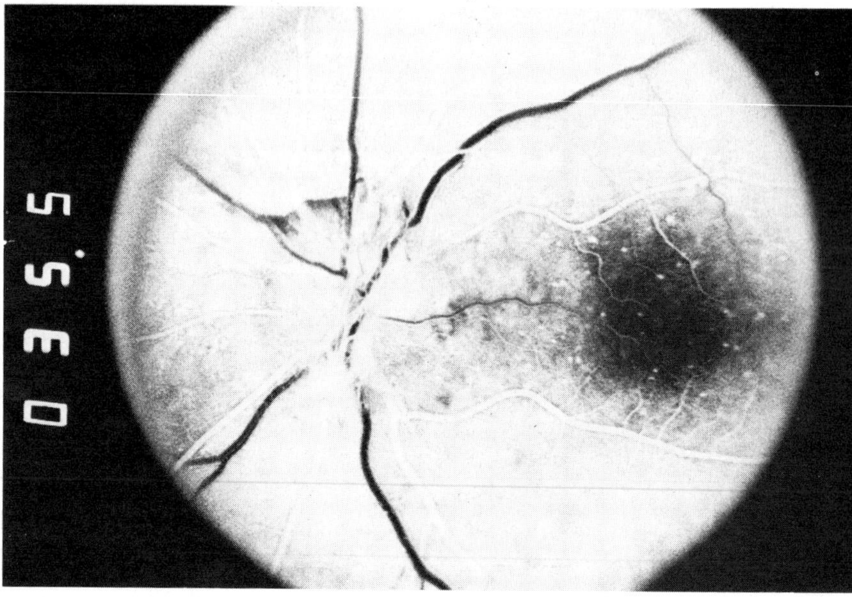

Fig. 7.34. Five seconds later, there is still no venous filling, demonstrating marked delay in intraretinal transit time.

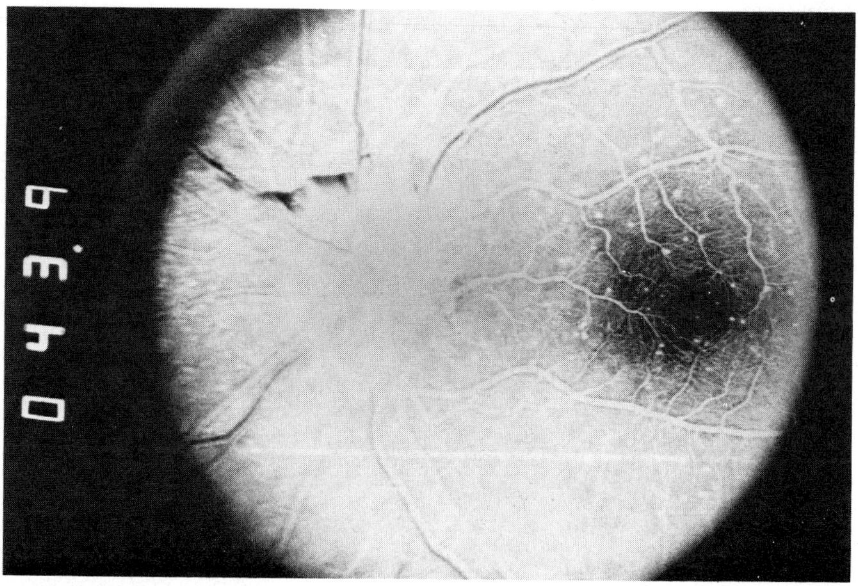

Fig. 7.35. When the capillary bed finally does fill, no microaneurysms are seen. Small, white dots seen in the fundus are drusen and are located at the level of the pigment epithelium. This was more easily appreciated on review of the photographs stereoscopically.

previous history of cerebrovascular accident and myocardial infarction. Ocular examination revealed vision of 20/70 O.D. and 20/80 O.S. Slit lamp examination was unremarkable. Fundus examination of the right eye demonstrated scattered microaneurysms. Fundus examination of the left eye demonstrated extensive optic disc neovascularization and a small preretinal hemorrhage inferior to the vascular arcades (Figures 7.32). The patient was diagnosed as having proliferative diabetic retinopathy and underwent fluorescein angiography which demonstrated marked delay in arterial perfusion and a marked delay in retinal transit time in the left eye (Figure 7.33–7.35).

This picture was consistent with marked ischemic oculopathy as the cause of the neovascularization, rather than diabetic microangiopathy. Three days after her examination, the patient lost vision in her left eye to no light perception and was found to have an ischemic infarct of the left optic nerve. Patient was admitted to the hospital, where a four-vessel arteriogram revealed a complete occlusion of the left internal carotid artery (Figure 7.36). Subtraction film of the orbit revealed collateral flow from the left external carotid into the ophthalmic artery, with retrograde flow into the cerebral circulation. The patient underwent reimplantation of the left vertebral into the left common carotid artery. She recovered from the operation and was followed as an out-patient. She did not regain vision in the left eye.

The patient was initially misdiagnosed as having proliferative retinopathy. The fluorescein angiogram demonstrated marked delay in perfusion and was instrumental in elucidating the correct diagnosis of ischemic oculopathy. It also raises the issue, again, of association between anterior ischemic optic neuropathy and carotid disease.

DISCUSSION

This potpourri of cases shows the many manifestations that extra-ocular vascular disease can bring to bear on the eye. Two of the patients were misdiagnosed as having macular edema, when they actually had impending central retinal artery obstruction. Perhaps earlier fluorescein angiography would have clarified the diagnosis, at least in one patient (Case IV). In the branch artery occlusion and the apparent cilioretinal artery occlusion, more widespread vascular pathology was suggested by the angiogram and was confirmed by subsequent arteriography. The patients with acute ischemic optic neuropathy (Cases V and VI) raise the issue of how much carotid artery disease contributes to posterior ciliary disease, either through embolization or hypoperfusion. And finally, a case of severe ocular hypoperfusion was seen to be causing retinal neovascularization, which was misdiagnosed as proliferative diabetic retinopathy.

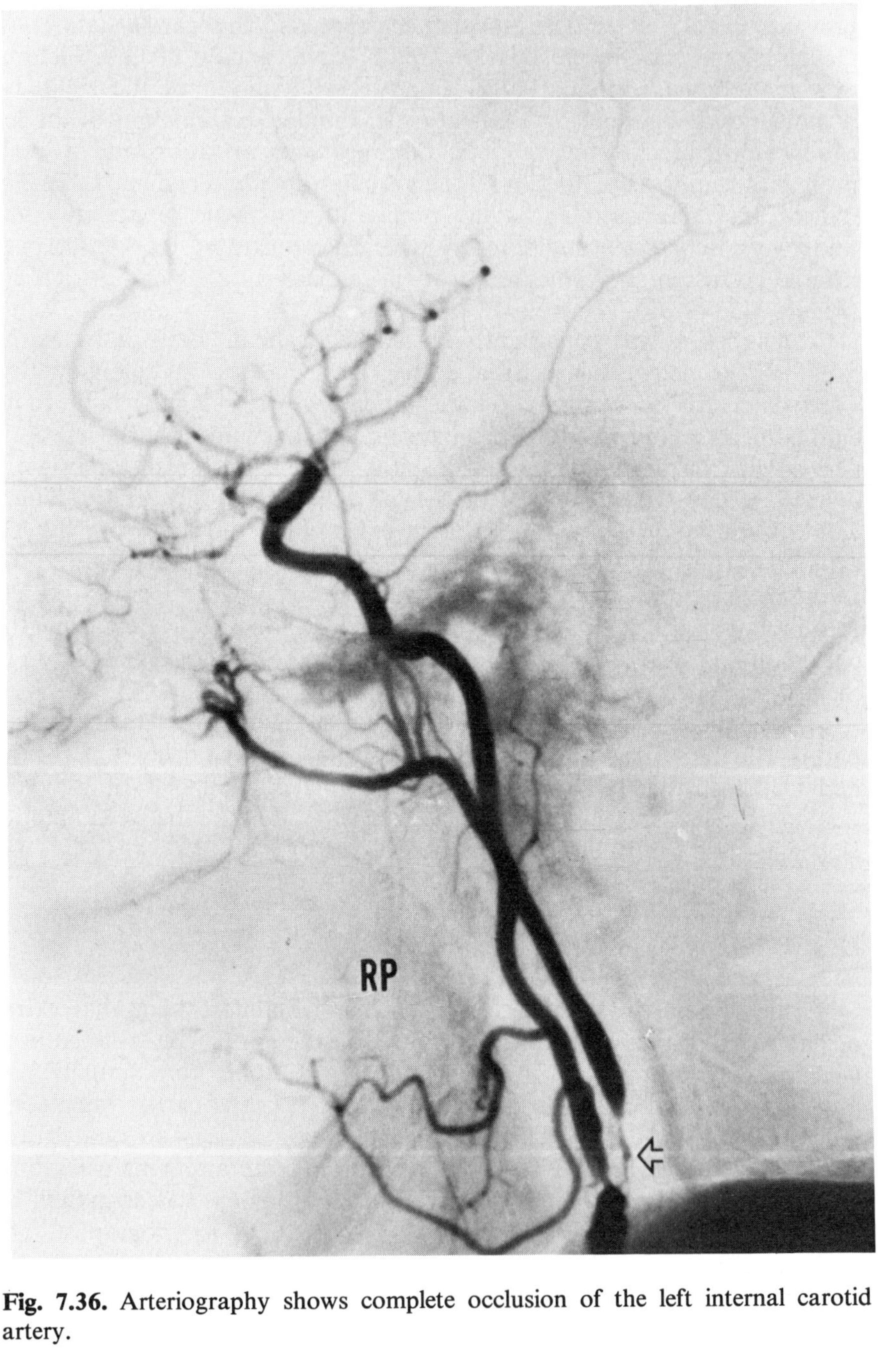

Fig. 7.36. Arteriography shows complete occlusion of the left internal carotid artery.

TABLE 7.1. Ocular ischemia syndromes

Acute	Chronic
Arterial occlusion central or branch	"Venous stasis"
Complete or impending ischemic optic neuropathy	Cotton wool spots
	Unilateral glaucoma
	Chronic uveitis
	Retinal neovascularization
	Iris neovascularization
	Orbital pain

These patients represent a few of the so-called ocular ischemia syndromes (Table 7.1). For convenience, these syndromes can be classified into acute or chronic, as illustrated in Table 7.1. The variety of syndromes and their multiplicity and also the high frequency with which they are seen certainly warrants close collaboration between ophthalmologists, vascular surgeons and neuroradiologists and closer attention to the pathology of the orbital vasculature as well as the extraorbital vasculature.

Fluorescein angiography is a common tool widely used by ophthalmologists. Ophthalmologists should be aware that this common test may often provide information about the status of the orbital vasculature as well as the carotid system; and that not only should we focus on the microvascular system of the retina when we look at a fluorescein angiogram, but we should be aware of macrovascular events as well. Heightened awareness of a normal arterial perfusion time, normal transit time, normal venous phases, and normal timing events will enrich the value of fluorescein angiography and allow us to detect pathology which previously has been overlooked.

REFERENCES

1. Novotny, H.R., and Alvis, D.L.: A method of photographing fluorescence in circulatory blood in the human retina. *Circulation* 24:82, 1961.
2. Hollenhorst, R.W., and Kearns, T.P.: Fluorescein dye test of circulation time in patients with occlusive disease of the carotid arterial system. *Proc. Mayo Clin.* 36:457, 1961.
3. David, N.J., Saito,Y., and Heyman, A.: Arm to retina fluorescein appearance time. *Arch. Neurol.* (Chicago) 5:165, 1961.
4. Pemberton, J.W., and Britton, W.A.: The arm-retina circulation time. *Arch. Ophthalmol.* 71:364, 1964.
5. David, N.J., Norton, E.W.C., Gass, J.D., and Sexton, R.: Fluorescein retinal angiography in carotid occlusion. *Arch. Neurol.* 14:281, 1966.
6. Newsom, W.A., Leverett, S.D., and Kirkland, V.E.: Fluorescein angiography and experimental carotid occlusion. *Arch. Ophthalmol.* 80:377, 1968.

8

CAROTID ARTERY DISEASE AND THE EYE

Larry E. Magargal, M.D.
George E. Sanborn, M.D*

Carotid artery disease can produce a variety of ocular and nonocular manifestations. The ocular manifestations are of importance not only because they occur in a high proportion of patients with carotid insufficiency (1), but because they are often the first indication that such carotid artery disease exists.

In general, patients with carotid artery disease present to the ophthalmologist in several different ways (2). Some patients have had a transient ischemic attack (TIA). When the TIA involves the carotid system, the symptoms include hemiparesis, hemisensory loss, aphasia or dysphasia, and transient monocular blindness (amaurosis fugax). The second group of patients have symptoms which are purely ocular: they include partial or complete visual loss due to an artery obstruction and decreased vision or pain resulting from the ocular ischemic syndrome. The third group of patients are asymptomatic and any ocular findings consistent with carotid artery disease are incidental.

GROUP I

Amaurosis Fugax

The type of TIA found in the first group of patients is the most common symptom of carotid artery disease (1). It is a sudden, painless, monocular loss of vision which typically lasts between two and ten minutes.

From the Retinal Vascular Unit, Wills Eye Hospital, Philadelphia, Pennsylvania.

*Dr. Sanborn is presently at the University of Utah Medical Center, Salt Lake City, Utah.

The patient frequently describes his vision as "dark" or "dim." The return of vision can be sectorial or altitudinal and is occasionally described as a "curtain rising." Generally the vision returns to normal immediately after an attack. The frequency of these attacks can vary from one or two attacks per month to 10 or 20 per day.

The retina, if observed during an amaurotic attack, may either be normal (3), show complete occlusion, exhibit migratory white retinal emboli within the retinal arterioles along with accompanying disruption of the arterial circulation (4), or demonstrate cholesterol emboli moving through the arterial system (3). The importance of recognizing amaurosis fugax as a TIA is that it is virtually always associated with serious atheromatous ulcerative disease of either the ipsilateral common carotid artery or the extracranial portion of the internal carotid artery, or both (5). Microembolization from this ulcerative lesion is the mechanism responsible for the amaurosis (6). Approximately one-third of all patients with an untreated TIA can be expected to have a stroke, a rate approximately four times the incidence in an age-matched population (7).

GROUP II

The second group of patients exhibit purely ocular symptoms. These patients may present with any form of retinal artery obstruction which is due to embolization originating from ulcerative atheroma in the carotid artery of the neck. The obstruction may be limited to sudden occlusion of either a branch artery, a cilioretinal artery, the central retinal artery, or the ophthalmic artery.

Venous Stasis Retinopathy

The appearance of chronic ophthalmic artery obstruction produced by hypoperfusion due to progressive stenosis of the ipsilateral internal carotid artery or the common carotid artery is characteristic. This condition is known as venous stasis retinopathy (8,9) or more appropriately, hypoperfusion retinopathy (10). Venous stasis retinopathy is not a good term for this condition because the basic mechanism involves reduction of the arterial inflow, not the venous outflow; even more confusion has resulted from the use of the term to describe the features of the nonischemic form of central retinal vein obstruction (11).

Hypoperfusion Retinopathy

Hypoperfusion retinopathy is characterized by dot and blot hemorrhages in the mid-periphery of the fundus, venous tortuosity and engorgement, microaneurysms, and areas of capillary nonperfusion. The condition does not usually affect the posterior pole although macular edema, when it is occasionally present, does produce a mild decrease in visual acuity. The entire 360° range of the eye is usually affected, although there may be more hemorrhages in one quadrant than another.

Ocular Ischemic Syndrome

In some cases carotid artery obstruction can lead to the ocular ischemic syndrome (12–14). In contrast to hypoperfusion retinopathy, which can result from unilateral carotid disease, the ocular ischemic syndrome is usually associated with bilateral carotid artery disease, although the syndrome can be unilateral or asymmetrical. The ocular ischemic syndrome is characterized posteriorly by hypoperfusion retinopathy and choroidal perfusion defects with some cases exhibiting neovascularization of either the disc or the retina elsewhere. Anteriorly there may be episcleral vascular congestion and signs of anterior segment ischemia which can consist of corneal edema, anterior chamber cells and flare (ischemic uveitis), neovascularization of the iris, elevated intraocular pressure, neovascular glaucoma, a poorly reactive pupil, and often severe orbital pain (ocular angina). The ischemic pain which can be seen is different from the pain secondary to elevated pressure due to neovascular glaucoma. Moreover, an embolic central retinal artery or branch retinal artery obstruction can occur in cases with subtotal carotid disease and can also occur in cases with the ocular ischemic syndrome because of circulatory stagnation.

GROUP III

The third group of patients are asymptomatic; signs of carotid artery disease are an incidental finding. Generally this incidental finding involves the discovery of retinal microemboli. These microemboli can be found in association with arterial obstructions, usually involving a branch of the central retinal artery. They are sometimes observed after or during an episode of amaurosis fugax (4).

Cholesterol Emboli

Two types of microemboli are associated with carotid artery disease. Cholesterol emboli are bright yellow or orange, often irregular in shape and slightly larger than the blood column; they are called Hollenhorst or bright plaques. They tend to lodge at the bifurcation of medium and small vessels, but can change position, moving downstream from one bifurcation to another. They generally do not produce a complete retinal artery obstruction, but can produce a localized partial obstruction of the arteriole which usually manifests as a dilation of the adjacent vein (15). Transient obstructions producing amaurosis fugax are common (16). Some of these emboli remain unchanged for long periods of time while others disappear. In some patients, an inflammatory segmental perivascular cuff will slowly appear at the site of a cholesterol lipid embolus, sometimes even obscuring the embolus (15). At times, fluorescein angiography will demonstrate evidence of microembolization after the embolus has disappeared under the ophthalmoscope (17).

Cholesterol emboli are caused by ulceration of an atheromatous lesion in the extracranial carotid artery. While such emboli have generally been felt to occur only when the extracranial carotid artery is not completely occluded, embolization distal to a completely occluded carotid artery has been documented (18), as has embolization from the external carotid artery (19).

Platelet–fibrin Emboli

Platelet–fibrin emboli are the second type of emboli associated with carotid artery disease. These emboli are greyish-white amorphous structures which are approximately the same sizes as the blood column. They are highly mobile, tending to move rapidly from one bifurcation to another, and to fragment quickly. They can be asymptomatic but may result in either an amaurosis fugax attack (4) or a branch retinal artery obstruction (16). Because of their fleeting nature, platelet–fibrin emboli are seen less often than cholesterol emboli (16). These emboli are composed predominantly of platelet aggregates and often orginate from an ulcerative lesion of the extracranial carotid artery (20).

Calcific Emboli

The third type of microemboli which can be seen in the retinal circulation is not associated with carotid artery disease, but typically originates from aortic or valvular heart disease (21). These are calcific emboli which are grey-white in color, the same size or larger than the arterial lumen, and are usually found near the optic disc. They frequently produce a high grade, sustained retinal artery occlusion.

Atheromata

A fourth type of intraluminal plaque within the arterial system is not an embolus; however, it is sometimes confused with one of the emboli previously described. This plaque is an atheroma involving the retinal arterioles. In the one case documented histopathologically, one eye was normal, but the other eye showed multiple yellow-white plaques which involved all of the retinal arteriole branches (22). The patient in this case had no evidence of extracranial carotid artery disease.

The importance of finding either cholesterol emboli or platelet–fibrin emboli within the eye has been well established. One study showed that 69% of patients with cholesterol emboli had either a TIA or a stroke within ten days of being examined (23). The increased incidence of stroke in patients with cholesterol or platelet–lipid emboli has been well documented (24); however, the largest single cause of death in these patients is not stroke but rather cardiovascular disease (25).

DIAGNOSIS

In addition to a complete history and ocular examination, the status of the extracranial carotid artery should be ascertained. Each carotid should be palpated and judged as to the strength of the pulse. This is important because the carotid pulse is often diminished or absent in the presence of a complete or near complete occlusion. Auscultation of the carotid should also be performed. The occurrence of a cervical bruit is related to extracranial carotid artery stenosis (26). The absence of a cervical bruit, however, does not mean that a significant stenotic lesion is not present (27). A bruit may be present in patients with high grade carotid obstruction, but may disappear when the carotid artery becomes completely occluded.

The best test for carotid artery disease is selective four vessel carotid arteriography, which employs an arterial injection of contrast material. However, this test is expensive, time consuming, and has a low but definite morbidity and mortality rate (28). Recently, digital subtraction angiography has been used in the diagnosis of carotid artery disease (29). With this technique, an intravenous catheter is introduced into the superior vena cava where contrast material is then injected. The images produced have bone and soft tissue structures subtracted and can be stored on video tape for replaying.

Digital subtraction angiography, when performed intravenously, however, has some disadvantages. Both carotid vessels and vertebral vessels are imaged at the same time. Thus it is difficult to obtain a true lateral of the carotid birfurcation without the opposite carotid being superimposed. The image quality is not quite as good as with selective intraarterial injection of contrast. On the other hand, the digital subtraction technique can be used in conjunction with selective intraarterial catheter injection (30) to provide improved imaging of a selected carotid artery from any angle. This can be done simply by performing a digital study using intravenous injection of contrast material. If this study shows an abnormality that needs further visualization, the intravenous catheter is removed from the arm and a percutaneous intraarterial catheter is inserted through the femoral artery. A selective study of any particular vessel can then be performed. This selective testing allows the procedure to be done faster, with less contrast material, and more safely than with conventional arteriography.

It is very likely that intraarterial selective contrast angiography will be performed in the future using the digital subtraction technique. The role of intravenous angiography using the digital subtraction technique, however, is unclear.

Noninvasive Testing

In order to avoid many of the problems inherent in conventional selective arteriography, a variety of techniques have been developed or modified for use in carotid artery disease testing. Generally these tests have been used for screening. Patients who have signs or symptoms of carotid artery disease, and who are surgical candidates, should have a definitive study which will best visualize both the extracranial carotid arteries and the intracranial circulation. Patients who are not surgical candiates have no need of invasive studies since the extent or nature of their carotid disease will have no bearing on their medical management.

The ideal screening test should be noninvasive, inexpensive, easy to perform (ideally without requiring highly trained personnel), easy to interpret, and have a high degree of sensitivity and specificity. The noninvasive tests which have been developed can basically be divided into two groups, indirect and direct.

The indirect tests are based on measurement or assessment of the carotid blood flow or pressure. The most common indirect tests include ophthalmodynamometry (ODM), oculophlethysmography (OPG), oculopneumoplethysmography (OPPG), and the periorbital Doppler. However, all of these tests have one problem in common; they cannot be used to detect a carotid artery stenosis of less than 80%. Experimental studies, as predicted by fluid mechanics, have verified that there is no significant pressure drop in the carotid artery distal to an obstruction until the diameter of the lumen of the vessel in reduced by at least 80%: the "critical stenosis" (31–33).

In the literature a number of studies overcome this testing problem by describing a particular technique which is very effective in identifying vessels with a high degree of stenosis. There is no evidence, however, that the degree of stenosis of the carotid artery has any correlation with the symptoms; indeed, there are a number of good clinical studies which suggest that such is not the case (27, 34, 35). Thus patients with ulcerative but nonstenotic lesions of the carotid are as likely to develop a stroke as those who have significant stenotic lesions.

The second group of tests are those which directly examine the carotid bifurcation. Theoretically tests that directly image the carotid should overcome the limitations of indirect tests since they do not depend on blood flow. However, they must be able to provide high quality imaging in order to detect small ulcerative lesions. These tests all provide information about a small portion of the extracranial carotid artery and no information at all about the intracranial circulation.

The three direct imaging methods are B-scan ultrasound, Doppler imaging without frequency analysis, and Doppler imaging with frequency analysis. Duplex scanning involves imaging the carotid with B-scan ultrasonography and then applying Doppler frequency analysis to this image. Duplex scanning appears to be the most sensitive test available for detecting lesions of the carotid which are both stenotic and nonstenotic. However, this technique requires expensive equipment and skilled personnel, both in performing the test and interpreting the results. It does not appear to qualify as a routine screening test. Whether this test will replace or substitute for digital subtraction angiography, either intravenous or intraarterial, will depend on future studies in which the two techniques are compared.

TREATMENT

The vascular surgical techniques for carotid artery disease is beyond the scope of this work. However, in general, if a patient is a surgical candidate and has an ulcerative or a hemodynamcially significant but not totally occluded lesion of the extracranial artery, an endarterectomy is the procedure of choice (36). For patients with a totally occluded carotid artery, a bypass procedure such as the superficial temporal artery—middle cerebral artery bypass is usually indicated (37).

For patients who are not surgical candidates, treatment with a platelet-antiaggregating agent in indicated. The evidence to date suggests that no agent or combination of agents is superior to the use of aspirin, although the optimal aspirin dosage has not yet been agreed upon (38).

In most cases, the decision regarding treatment for a particular patient with carotid artery disease will be made by a vascular surgeon, a neurologist, or a neurosurgeon. However, the ophthalmologist will be involved in the recognition and treatment of patients with the ocular ischemic syndrome. In our experience, the aggressive treatment of the ocular ischemic syndrome can result in stabilization of vision, relief of ocular pain, and in some cases, improved vision.

The first step in the treatment of glaucoma resulting from the ocular ischemic syndrome is to treat neovascular glaucoma if it is present. While this is initially treated with oral and topical agents, combined angle and panretinal photocoagulation are useful in cases without complete secondary angle closure. With complete angle closure, cyclocryotherapy is usually necessary. If the ischemic drive can be reduced and the angle maintained, the prognosis for maintaining useful vision is increased.

In the event that visualization of the fundus is impossible because of a cataract or other media opacities, a peripheral retinal cryoablation provides a simple alternative to panretinal photocoagulation. In addition to reducing the ischemic drive, an attempt is made to improve the ophthalmic artery circulation through a surgical procedure. Both carotid endarterectomy (39) and carotid artery bypass surgery (40) have been effective in increasing perfusion to the eye. After vascular surgery is performed, the signs of anterior segment ischemia frequently decrease and patients may experience a striking relief of ocular pain. After the eye has stabilized, cataract surgery may be necessary in order to improve visual acuity.

SUMMARY

Carotid artery disease commonly presents with a variety of ocular signs and symptoms which can be divided into either embolic or hypoperfusion effects. The ophthalmologist is frequently in a unique position to make the diagnosis and institute appropriate studies. Prompt recognition of the presence of carotid artery disease allows for the improved ocular, vascular, and medical treatment that is available today.

ACKNOWLEDGMENT

Supported in part by the Retina Research and Development Foundation, Philadelphia, Pennsylvania and The Lions Fight for Sight Conservation, Incorporated, Pennsylvania.

REFERENCES

1. Hollenhorst, R.W.: Ocular manifestations of insufficiency or thrombosis of the internal carotid artery. *Am. J. Ophthalmol.* 47:753, 1959.
2. Henkind, P., and Chambers, J.K.: Arterial occlusive disease of the retina. In Duane, T.D., Jaeger, E.A., eds. *Clinical Ophthalmology*, vol. 2. Philadelphia: Harper & Row, 1982, Chapter 14, pp. 1–14.
3. Hollenhorst, R.W.: The neuro-ophthalmology of strokes. In Smith J.L., ed. *Neuro-ophthalmology*. vol II. St. Louis: C.V. Mosby, 1965, pp.100-121.

4. Fisher, M.C.: Observation of the fundus oculi in transient monocular blindness. *Neurology* 9:333, 1959.
5. Sandok, B.A., Trautmann, J.C., Ramirez-Lassepas, M., Sundt, T.M., and Houser, O.W.: Clinical-angiographic correlations in amaurosis fugax. *Am. J. Ophthalmol.* 79:137, 1974.
6. Kearns, T.P.: Ophthalmology and the carotid artery. *Am. J. Ophthalmol.* 88:714, 1979.
7. Goldner, J.C., Whisnant, J.P., and Taylor, W.F.: Long-term prognosis of transient cerebral ischemic attacks. *Stroke* 2:160, 1971.
8. Hedges, T.R.: Ophthalmoscopic findings in internal carotid artery occlusion. *Bull. Johns Hopkins Hosp.* 3:89, 1962.
9. Kearns, T.P., and Hollenhorst, R.W.: Venous-stasis retinopathy of occlusive disease of the carotid artery. Mayo clin Proc. 38:304, 1963.
10. Green, W.R.: Histopathologic studies of hypotensive retinopathy, branch vein occlusion, and central retinal vein occlusion. In Fine, S.L., and Owens, S.L., eds. *Management of Retinal Vascular and Macular Disorders.* Baltimore: Williams & Wilkins, 1982, pp. 5-27.
11. Hayreh, S.S.: So-called "central retinal vein occlusion." II. Venous stasis retinopathy. *Ophthalmologica* 172:14, 1976.
12. Knox, D.L.: Ischemic ocular inflammation. *Am. J. Ophthalmol.* 60:995, 1965.
13. Brown, G.C., Magargal, L.E., Simeone, F.A., Goldberg, R.E., Federman, J.L., and Benson, W.E.: Arterial obstruction and ocular neovascularization. *Ophthalmology* 89:139, 1982.
14. Gonder, J.R., Kiser,D., Sanborn, G.E., Magargal, L.E., and Simeone, F.: The ocular ischemic syndrome. An indication for neovascular surgery. *Ann. Royal Coll. Surg.* (Canada) 16:447, 1983.
15. Hoyt, W.F.: Ocular symptoms and signs. In: Wylie, E.J., Ehrenfeld, W.K., eds. *Extracranial Cerebrovascular Disease.* Diagnosis and Management. Philadelphia: W.B. Saunders, 1970, p. 64.
16. Arruga, J., and Sanders, M.D.: Ophthalmologic findings in 70 patients with evidence of retinal embolism. *Ophthalmology* 89:1336, 1982.
17. Muci-Mendoza, R., Arruga, J., Edwards, W.O., and Hoyt, W.F.: Retinal fluorescein evidence for atheromatous microembolism. *Stroke* 11:154, 1980.
18. Countee, R.W., Vijayanathan, T., and Chavis P.: Recurrent retinal ischemia beyond cervical carotid occlusions. Clinical-angiographic correlations and therapeutic implications. *J. Neurosurg.* 55:532, 1981.
19. Burnbaum, M.D., Selhorst, J.B., Harbison, J.W., and Brush, J.J.: Amaurosis fugax from disease of the external carotid artery. *Arch. Neurol.* 34:532, 1977.
20. McBrien, D.J., Bradley, R.D., and Ashton, N.: The nature of retinal emboli in stenosis of the internal carotid artery. *Lancet* 1:697, 1963.
21. Ross Russell, R.W.: The source of retinal emboli. *Lancet* 2:789, 1968.
22. Brownstein, S., Font, R.L., and Alper, M.G.: Atheromatous plaques of the retinal blood vessels. Histologic confirmation of ophthalmoscopically visible lesions. *Arch. Ophthalmol.* 1973;90:49-52.
23. Hollenhorst, R.W.: Vascular status of patients who have cholesterol emboli in the retina. *Am J. Ophthalmol.* 61:1159/219-1165/225, 1966.
24. Pfaffenbach, D.D., and Hollenhorst, R.W.: Morbidity and Survivorship of patients with embolic cholesterol crystals in the ocular fundus. *Am. J. Ophthalmol.* 75:66, 1973.
25. Savino, P.J., Glaser, J.S., and Cassady, J.: Retinal stroke. Is the patient at risk? *Arch. Ophthalmol.* 95:1185, 1977.
26. Riles, T.S., Lieberman, A., Kopelman, I., and Imparato, A.M.: Symptoms, stenosis, and bruit. Interrelationships in carotid artery disease. *Arch. Surg.* 116:218, 1981.

27. David, T.E., Humphries, A.W., Young, J.R., and Beven, E.G.: A correlation of neck bruits and arteriosclerotic carotid arteries. *Arch. Surg.* 107:729, 1973.
28. Faught, E., Trader, S.D., and Hannah, G.R.: Cerebral complications of angiography for transient ischemia and stroke: prediction of risk. *Neurology* 29:4, 1979.
29. Brody, W.R., Enzmann, D.R., Miller, D.C., Guthaner, D.F., Pelc, N.J., Keyes, G.S., and Riederer, S.J.: Intravenous arteriography using digital subtraction techniques. *JAMA* 248:671, 1982.
30. Forbes, G.S., Ernest, F., Kispert, D.B., Folger, W.N., and Sundt, T.M.: Digital angiography. Introducing digital techniques to clinical cerebral angiography practice. *Mayo Clin. Proc.* 57:683, 1982.
31. Mann, F.C., Herrick, J.F., Essex, H.E., and Balder, E.J.: The effect on the blood flow of decreasing the lumen of a blood vessel. *Surgery* 4:249, 1938.
32. Rand, R.W.: Retinal arterial pressure studies associated with cervical carotid artery occlusion in the treatment of cerebral aneurysms. Bull. Los Angeles Neurol. Soc. 21:175, 1956.
33. May, A.G., DeWeese, J.A., and Rob, C.G.: Hemodynamic effects of arterial stenosis. *Surgery* 53:513, 1963.
34. Thiele, B.L., Young, J.V., Chikos, P.M., Hirsh, J.H., and Strandness, D.E.: Correlation of arteriographic findings and symptoms in cerebrovascular disease. *Neurology* 30:1041, 1980.
35. Dyken, M.L., Klatte, E., Kolar, O.J., and Spurgeon, C.: Complete occlusion of common or internal carotid arteries. *Arch. Neurol.* 30:343, 1974.
36. Allen, G.S., and Preziosi, T.J.: Carotid endarterectomy: a prospective study of its efficacy and safety. *Medicine* 60:298, 1981.
37. Kearns, T.P., Siekert, R.G., and Sundt, T.M.: The ocular aspects of bypass surgery of the carotid artery. *Mayo Clin. Proc.* 54:3, 1979.
38. Dyken, M.L.: Anticoagulant and platelet-antiaggregating therapy in stroke and threatened stroke. *Neurol. Clin.* 1:223, 1983.
39. Neupert, J.R., Brubaker, R.F., Kearns, T.P., and Sundt, T.M.: Rapid resolution of venous stasis retinopathy after carotid endarterectomy. *Am. J. Ophthalmol.* 81:600, 1976.
40. Kearns, T.P., Younge, B.R., and Piepgras, D.G.: Resolution of venous stasis retinopathy after carotid artery bypass surgery. *Mayo Clin. Proc.* 55:342, 1980.

9

ANTERIOR SEGMENT ISCHEMIA OF THE EYE

Robert S. Jampel, M.D., Ph.D
John M. Ramocki, M.D.

The eye is divided into an anterior and a posterior segment. The anterior segment contains the refractive mechanisms and the posterior segment the sensory mechanisms. The two segments are considered to have two separate but overlapping blood supplies. This paper is a brief review of the vascular diseases associated with the anterior segment and their possible relationship to the diseases of the carotid arteries. It should be made clear at the onset that little is specifically known concerning the vascular diseases of the anterior segment of the eye and their relationship to systemic diseases or to the diseases of the anterior part of the eye: presbyopia, cataract, glaucoma, uveitis, and age related degeneration. Also, little is known about the relationship between carotid artery disease and anterior segment vascular disease.

CHARACTERISTICS OF THE ANTERIOR SEGMENT

Circulation

The entire eyeball and orbital contents are supplied by the ophthalmic artery, a major branch of the internal carotid artery. There is, however, a collateral blood supply by means of the infraorbital artery and the middle meningeal artery which are branches of the external carotid artery. This ancillary or secondary supply may be activated when the primary system is impaired.

From the Kresge Eye Institute of Wayne State University, Detroit, Mi.

The blood supply of the anterior segment of the eye is derived from the two long posterior ciliary arteries and the seven anterior ciliary arteries. The anterior ciliaries are derived from the lacrimal or second branch of the ophthalmic artery and the long posteriors from the ciliary or third branch of the ophthalmic artery. The long posterior ciliary arteries pass forward in the suprachoroidal space on the medial and lateral sides of the eye before bifurcating several millimeters posterior to the limbal margin to form deep paralimbal branches. These paralimbal branches are responsible for the formation of the major arterial circle and provide vessels which supply the ciliary muscle, stroma and processes. There are no anastomoses between the anterior ciliaries and the major arterial circle in humans according to Woodlief (1) although these are shown in diagrams in a major textbook (2). Precapillary sphincters have been demonstrated at the branch points of the arterioles to the ciliary processes. These suggest the presence of a mechanism for controlling blood supply to the capillaries of the ciliary processes and, therefore, controlling aqueous humor production (1).

The anterior ciliary arteries run forward in variable locations on the tendons of the rectus muscles usually two on each tendon except for the lateral rectus which has only one (3). After penetrating the sclera they bifurcate at the root of the iris to form deep paralimbal branches which give off capillary networks supplying the ciliary body and radial branches, which in turn pass under the major arterial circle, to supply the iris. Superficial networks derived from nonpenetrating branches of the anterior ciliary arteries anastomose with deep networks to supply the perilimbal conjunctiva, the episclera and Schlemm's Canal. The capillary bed of the ciliary processes has a diffusing surface of about seven square centimeters (2).

Collateral circulation occurs at three interconnecting sites in the anterior segment: the episcleral circle, the intramuscular circle, and the major arterial circle. The episcleral circle is composed of anastomosing superficial capillary networks derived from the anterior ciliaries. The intermuscular circle is formed by anastomosing capillary networks given off by the perforating anterior ciliaries and the long posteriors. It is the most extensive of the three interconnected arterial rings. The major arterial circle is derived from the long posterior ciliaries, and is frequently discontinuous. The anterior choroidal vessels also contribute blood to the anterior segment and indirectly to the major arterial circle. These vascular circles account for the rarity of anterior segment ischemia following most types of ophthalmic surgery (3).

Microdissection and scanning electron microscopy of primate ocular vascular castings and iris angiography have helped to delineate the vasculature of the anterior segment. There is a segmental and an irregular filling pattern of the iris, a blood–iris barrier and a rudimentary minor arterial circle at the level of the collarette where a loose meshed and sparse capillary network is formed. On reaching the pupil these arterioles resolve into well-formed capillary networks and then collect into a system of venules that course deep to the arteries on their way to the ciliary body and the vortex veins (4).

Little is understood concerning the regulation of the anterior segment circulation. The retina appears autoregulated, but the uvea is influenced by chemical and nervous stimuli. The effects of prostaglandins, alpha receptors, cholinergic substances, and various other chemicals and drugs have yet to be clarified (5). Retinal vascular occlusions can cause anterior segment ischemia. How this occurs is not known. Perfusion deficiencies of the anterior segment are often found shortly after an occlusive episode of the posterior segment and long before rubeosis develops. Some acute mechanism appears to be present that causes a circulatory redistribution that deprives the anterior segment of blood for the sake of survival of the retina. Redistribution of blood is known to result from choroidal vasodilation and simultaneous constriction of the ciliary body and iris vessels. This results in the siphoning of blood away from the anterior segment and into the posterior uvea (4).

Fluorescein angiography of the anterior segment is to date the only available method that shows promise in the diagnosis and investigation of the circulation in the anterior segment. The vertical anterior ciliary arteries, for example, appear to be especially important to anterior segment blood flow. This is demonstrated by high incidence of delayed filling of the inferotemporal iris quadrant and of temporal iris atrophy following vertical muscle surgery (6). Also, fluorescein angiography has demonstrated anterior segment perfusion defects and iris vascular leakage in all patients tested who had Fuch's heterochromic cyclitis (7). Thus it follows that chronic ischemia is an integral part of this disease process and helps explain the rubeosis and neovascular glaucoma associated with this disease. Iris angiography (4) has demonstrated abnormalities in the blood flow of the anterior segment associated with essential iris atrophy, uveitis, posterior segment vascular disease, rubeosis and neovascular glaucoma, macular edema, and retinitis pigmentosa (4).

Structure Of The Vessels Of The Anterior Segment

The structure of the vessels of the anterior segment of the eye has never been systematically studied and information is sparse (2). The ciliary vessels are typical small arteries with an endothelial lining surrounded by intima, a media of smooth muscle fibers, and an adventitia of collagen. The major arterial circle has an endothelium with a distinct basement membrane, media with two or three layers of smooth muscle cells and adventitia with loose collagenous tissue. The capillaries of the ciliary processes are large and have a thin fenestrated endothelium which is permeable to myoglobin. The vessels of the iris are unique. They are corkscrew in shape and have a thick, collagenous, circularly oriented adventitia separated from the endothelium by a less dense space containing fewer fibrils and ground substance than usual. The muscle layer is interrupted.

CLINICAL AND EXPERIMENTAL WORK

The first description of anterior segment ischemia was by Schmidt in 1874 (8). His early cases were the result of bilateral arterial occlusion of the upper extremities, head, and neck which were associated with a diffuse ischemic oculopathy. Posterior segment changes were present along with anterior segment involvement. These accounts provided a description of a clinical syndrome. However, interest was centered mainly on the changes in the posterior segment (9).

In 1941, Leinfelder and Black (10) listed a number of eye complications following experimental transposition of the extraocular muscles in monkeys. They noted mild iridocyclitis, one case of heminecrosis of the iris, and a persistent dilation of the pupil. The association between vascular compromise and these signs was not clear. Lindner (11) advised against cutting more than two muscles at a time during retinal detachment surgery. Several case reports of postoperative anterior segment ischemia followed: iridocyclitis occurring postoperatively after a muscle transposition (12); heminecrosis of the iris following surgery on a high myope (13); striate keratitis; a fixed eccentric pupil; white deposits on the anterior lens capsule; high compound astigmatism followed later by heminecrosis of the iris; and eccentric pupil after strabismus surgery (14). Kornbleuth (15) discovered that the rate of flow of the aqueous diminished following surgery on the rectus muscles in rabbits. She believed that the decrease in rate of aqueous formation was due to severance of the anterior ciliary arteries. Evidence that extraocular muscle surgery could compromise the blood supply to the anterior segment was accumulating.

Girard in 1960 (16) removed and reinserted three or four rectus muscles from adult and infant monkeys. The adult monkeys developed chemosis of the conjuctiva, iridocyclitis, striate keratitis, necrosis of the iris, anterior cortical cataract, and hypotonia. Inflammation often subsided with steroid therapy but the complications developed and progressed despite treatment. Histopathology in one eye showed ischemic necrosis and atrophy of the iris, ciliary body, a segment of the anterior sclera, and the cornea. Acute and chronic iridocyclitis and keratitis and cataract and a fibrovascular membrane on the iris were also seen. Infant monkeys were not affected.

Wilson and Irvine (17) documented necrosis of the iris and ciliary body following retinal detachment surgery and Boniuk and Zimmerman in 1960 (18) reported three cases of necrosis of the iris and ciliary body followed scleral buckling with circling polyethylene tubes.

In 1966 Freeman (19) applied diathermy to both long ciliary arteries of the rabbit and produced corneal edema, hypotony, iris atrophy, cataracts, and phthisis bulbi. Cryoapplication to both arteries did not cause the syndrome. Crock (20) used the term anterior segment ischemia syndrome. He believed that milder forms of this syndrome were overlooked because of a latent period between the onset of ischemia and the appearance of signs in the anterior segment. Anderson (21) used diathermy of the long posterior ciliaries plus tenotomies of the rectus muscles to produce the anterior segment syndrome in albino rats in 1971. Muscle surgery alone was unable to produce this syndrome in rats.

Since most human eyes undergoing anterior segment surgery do not develop signs of ischemia, predisposing causes were sought. Von Noorden (22) attributed ischemia following an extraocular muscle operation to arteriosclerosis. Fells (23) reported ischemia following muscle surgery in patients with a history of contralateral carotid artery ligation. Jacobs (24) reported a case of anterior segment ischemia after muscle surgery in a patient with chronic lymphocytic leukemia. Fells and Marsh (25) reported ischemia in a dysthyroid patient after undergoing simultaneous recessions of adjacent inferior and medial rectus muscles.

Hiatt's 1977 (26) studies on dogs and monkeys indicated individual variations as to the susceptibility to the syndrome. He maintained that three or four recti should not be cut in adults at one operation, and that a three to six months interval between operations be allowed to enable collateral circulation to develop. The interval can be shorter in children (27).

ETIOLOGY

Any insult to the circulation of the anterior segment of the eye may cause ischemia. Vascular diseases involving the aorta, carotid arteries, ophthalmic arteries, and ciliary arteries may have effects on the capillary networks of the anterior segment and produce the signs of ischemia (28–31). No one has as yet correlated arteriosclerosis of the carotid arteries with vascular disease in the anterior segment.

The onset of the syndrome may be acute or insidious and its effects partial or complete. It may occur suddenly following extraocular muscle surgery of more than two muscles (16), traumatic occlusions or excessive diathermy of the long posterior ciliary arteries, strangulation of the long posteriors caused by pulling a scleral buckle too tight (32), or cryopexy or diathermy of the ciliary body in hemorrhagic glaucoma. Patients with hemoglobin SC disease (33, 34), arteriosclerosis, cardiac disease, malignant hypertension (35), diabetes, high myopia, and local ocular vascular disease are susceptible to developing the syndrome postoperatively. It may occur insidiously in vasculitis, uveitis, and during the aging process. It may be partial and segmental due to a scleral implant or focal vascular disease (32). In its complete form it may cause general infarction of the anterior segment which may ultimately lead to phthisis. Anterior segment necrosis with sloughing of the anterior part of the eye represents a disastrous outcome.

Anterior segment ischemia may result from or be associated with aortitis (28), carotid-cavernous fistula (36), temporal arteritis (37, 38), Buerger's disease, acute narrow angle glaucoma, orbital disease, infections, and irradiation.

Attempts to treat an ischemic syndrome with diathermy, laser coagulation, cryopexy or retrobulbar injection may exacerbate it by converting an anterior ischemia into an anterior segment necrosis if the vascular pathogenesis of the signs is not understood. This is evidenced by the case reports of anterior segment necrosis following treatment of a central retinal artery occlusion (39) and ischemic ocular necrosis from treatment of a carotid-cavernous fistula (36).

Diseases of the anterior segment in which ischemia may be a primary or contributing cause are listed below:

Cataract: Many theories exist as to the cause of cataract. The progression of lens opacification and vacuolization usually follows a chronic and intermittent course. The lens is an avascular organ surrounded by a clear fluid, the aqueous humor, which transmits substances to the lens to maintain its vitality. These substances diffuse through or are actively processed by the ciliary epithelium which is dependent on large fenestrated capillaries for its survival. The ciliary epithelium and capillaries form a diffusion surface of about seven square centimeters (2). It is reasonable to assume that damage to the ciliary capillary bed by sclerosis, vasculitis, or occlusive disease could have a deleterious effect on the composition of the aqueous humor. This in turn could produce lens opacification.

Glaucoma: Pathological vascular changes in the deep capillaries that supply the trabecular meshwork and Schlemm's canal could be responsible for the blockage of aqueous outflow. Conversely, ciliary body infarction could cause a decrease in aqueous formation resulting in hypotony.

Uveitis: Vascular damage resulting from occlusive disease or acute and chronic vascular immune reactions could be responsible for uveitis.

Aging: The degeneration and atrophy of ocular tissues associated with the aging process may be associated with arteriosclerosis.

In brief, the chronic diseases of the anterior segment of the eye may have significant associated vascular disease components, some of which may be related to general vascular disease and to diseases of the carotid arteries.

CLINICAL SYNDROME

The signs of anterior segment ischemia may be dramatic or subtle and involve all the tissues of the anterior segment (31). The conjunctiva may become hyperemic and chemotic. The cornea may develop diffuse epithelial and stromal edema. A cellular and protein response may be evident in the aqueous humor, indicating an inflammation of the iris and ciliary body. Large keratic precipitates may accumulate on the corneal endothelium causing damage to these cells. Recurrent corneal erosions and epithelial bullae may appear. A chronic stromal edema may eventually lead to interstitial neovascularization, dystrophic calcification and fatty infiltrations of the cornea.

Edema of the iridal stroma, stromal ecchymosis, or iridal cysts, either temporary or permanent may develop with or without broad bands of peripheral anterior synechiae. Segmental iridal necrosis with distortion of the pupil is a frequent finding. Rubeosis iridis with neovascular glaucoma may develop. Ectropion uvea may result from the contraction of an iris membrane. Severe ischemia can cause the eye to go on to phthisis bulbi or produce anterior segment necrosis with sloughing of the layer of the front of the eye.

Any layer of the lens may develop opacities, with flecks on the anterior capsule being the most common occurrence. These are often associated with the development of posterior synechiae. A mature cataract can develop over several months or over several days if the ischemia is severe.

Either hypotony or glaucoma may occur, with increased intraocular pressure not uncommon if neovascularization occurs. Severe ischemia may cause the eye to go on to phthisis bulbi or produce true anterior segment necrosis with sloughing of the layers of the front of the eye.

SUMMARY

Knowledge of the anatomy, physiology and pathology of the anterior segment of the eye is still rudimentary, but the importance of understanding the blood supply to the anterior part of the eye is now apparent. What was once described as an anterior segment necrosis occurring occasionally after extensive ophthalmic surgery is now understood as an anterior segment ischemic syndrome that manifests itself in a broad spectrum of signs and symptoms. Anterior segment ischemic syndrome can result in a severe necrosis of the anterior segment requiring enucleation on one end of the scale to a mild iridocyclitis recognized only by slit-lamp biomicroscopy on the other end. It may result from ophthalmic surgery or arteriosclerosis in the aging or be part of a systemic vascular disease. It may be related to a compromise in the blood supply to the head and neck or to a minimal defect in the blood vessels of the anterior segment of the eye that can be demonstrated only by iris angiography. ASIS can be associated with carotid artery disease, retinitis pigmentosa, central retinal artery or vein occlusion or Fuch's heterochromic cyclitis. It may play either a primary or secondary role in such common chronic diseases of the anterior segment as presbyopia, cataract, iritis, glaucoma, and corneal dystrophy.

The methods for study of the anterior circulation have yet to be perfected and this is an area for important clinical and basic research.

REFERENCES

1. Woodlief, N.F.: Initial observations on the ocular microcirculation in man. I. The anterior segment and extraocular muscles. *Arch. Ophthalmol.* 98:1268, 1980.
2. Hogan, M.J., Alvarado, A.B., and Weddell, J.E.: *Histology of the Human Eye.* Philadelphia: W.B. Saunders Co., 1971.
3. Morrison, J.C., and van Buskirk, M.D.: Anterior collateral circulation in the primate eye. *Ophthalmology,* 90:707, 1983.
4. Kottow, M.H.: Fluorescein angiography of the anterior segment. In: Peyman, *Principles of Ophthalmology,* Philadelphia: W.B. Saunders Co., 1980.
5. Bill, A.: Ocular circulation. In Moses, *Adler's Physiology of the Eye,* St. Louis: The C.V. Mosby Company, 1981.
6. Hayreh, S.S., and Scott, W.E.: Fluorescein iris angiography. II. Disturbances in iris circulation following strabismus operation on the various recti. *Arch. Ophthalmol.* 96:1390, 1978.
7. Berger, B.B., et al: Anterior segment ischemia in Fuch's heterochromic cyclitis. *Arch. Ophthalmol.* 98:499-501, 1980.
8. Schmidt, H.: Beitrag zur Kenntnis der Embolie der Anterior Centralis Retinae. *Arch. für Ophthal.* 20:287, 1874.
9. Kearns, T.P.: Ophthalmology and the carotid artery. *Am. J. Ophthalmol.* 88:714, 1979.
10. Leinfelder, P.J., and Black, N.M., Jr.: Experimental transposition of the extraocular muscles in monkeys. *Am. J. Ophthalmol.* 24:1115-1120, 1941.
11. Linder, J.: Ophthalmologische Operation Slehre. In Thiel, R., ed. Stuttgart, Germany: George Thieme Verlag, Vol. 2, 1945.
12. Stucchi, C., and Bianchi, F.: Depigmentation en secteur de consecutive a des transplantations musculaires. *Ophthalmologica,* 133:231, 1957.

13. Borley, W.E., and Synder, A.A.: Surgical treatment of high myopia: the combined lamellar scleral resection with scleral reinforcement, using donor eyes. *Trans. Am. Acad. Ophthalmol.* 62:791, 1958.
14. Forbes, S.B.: Muscle transplantation for external rectus paralysis; report of case with unusual complications. *Am. J. Ophthalmol.* 48:248, 1959.
15. Kornbleuth, W., et al: The effect of extraocular muscle surgery on aqueous humor dynamics. *Am. J. Ophthalmol.* 48:321, 1959.
16. Girard, L.J., and Beltranena, F.: Early and late complications of extensive muscle surgery. *Arch. Ophthalmol.* 64:576, 1960.
17. Wilson, W.A., and Irvine, S.R.: Pathologic changes following disruption of blood supply to iris and ciliary body. *Trans. Am. Acad. Ophthalmol. Otolaryngology* 59:501, 1955.
18. Boniuk, M. and Zimmerman, L.E.: Necrosis of the iris, ciliary body, lens, and retina following scleral buckling operations with circling polyethylene tubes. *Trans. Am. Acad. Ophthalmol. Otolaryngology* 65:671, 1961.
19. Freeman, H.M., Hawkins, W.R., and Schepens, C.L.: Anterior segment necrosis: an experimental study. *Arch. Ophthalmol.* 75:644, 1966.
20. Crock, G.: Clinical syndromes of anterior segment ischemia. *Trans. Ophthalmol. Soc. U.K.* 87:513, 1967.
21. Anderson, D.M., and Morin, J.D.: Experimental anterior segmental necrosis and rubeosis iridis. *Canad. J. Ophthalmol.* 6:196, 1971.
22. vonNoorden, G.K.: Anterior segment ischemia following the Jensen procedure. *Arch. Ophthalmol.* 94:845, 1976.
23. Fells, P.: Vertical rectus muscle transplantation to restore abduction in orthoptics. In Mein, J., Bierlaagh, J.J., and Brummelkamp-Dons, T.E.A. eds.: *Proceedings of the Second International Orthoptic Congress,* 1971, Amsterdam: Excerpta Medica, 1972, pp. 229-237.
24. Jacobs, D.S., Vastine, D.W., and Urist, M.J.: Anterior segent ischemia and sector iris atrophy after strabismus surgery in a patient with chronic lymphocytic leukemia. *Ophthalmol. Surg.* 7:42, 1976.
25. Fells, P., and Marsh, R.J.: Anterior segment ischemia following surgery on two rectus muscles. In Reinecke, R. D. ed., *Strabismus.* New York: Grune and Stratton, 1978, p. 375.
26. Hiatt, R.L.: Production of anterior segment ischemia. *Trans. Am. Ophthalmol. Soc.* 75:87, 1977.
27. Caputo, A.R., and Wagner, R.S.: Anterior segment ischemia following strabismus surgery. In Harley, *Pediatric Ophthalmology.* New York: Harper & Row, 1980.
28. Dowling, J.L., and Smith, T.R.: Ocular study of pulseless disease. *Arch. Ophthal.* 64:236, 1960.
29. Font, R.L., and Naumann, G.: Ocular Histopathology in pulseless disease. *Arch. Ophthalmol.* 82:784, 1969.
30. Michelson, P.E., Knox, D.L., and Green, W.R.: Ischemic ocular inflammation. *Arch. Ophthalmol.* 86:274, 1971.
31. Knox, D.L.: Ischemic ocular inflammation. *Am. J. Ophthalmol.* 60:995, 1965.
32. Robertson, D.M.: Anterior segment ischemia after segmental episcleral buckling and cryopexy. *Am. J. Ophthalmol.* 79:871, 1975.
33. Ryan, S.J., and Goldberg, M.F.: Anterior segment ischemia following scleral buckling in sickle cell hemoglobinopathy. *Am. J. Ophthalmol.* 72:35, 1971.
34. Eagle, R.C., Yanoff, M., and Morse, P.H.: Anterior segment necrosis following scleral buckling in hemoglobin SC disease. *Am. J. Ophthalmol.* 75:426, 1973.
35. deBuen, S., and Velazquez, T.: Ocular histopathology of malignant hypertension. *Sub. Rev. An. Soc. Mexicana Oftal.* 33:1, 1960.

36. Spencer, W.H., et al: Ischemic ocular necrosis from carotid cavernous fistula. *Br. J. Ophthalmol.* 57:145, 1973.
37. Spencer, W.H., and Hoyt, W.S.: A fatal case of giant cell arteritis with ocular involvement. *A.M.A. Arch. Ophthalmol.* 64:862, 1960.
38. Daicker, B., and Keller, H.: Giant cell arteritis with end ocular spreading and hypotonic bulbi dolorasa. *Klin. Monatbl. Augenheilkd.* 158:358, 1971.
39. Weidaw, C.D., et al: Anterior segment necrosis following treatment of central retinal artery occlusion. *Ann. Ophthalmol.* 199, 1978.

DISCUSSION: SESSION TWO

OCULOPLETHYSMOGRAPHY

Oculoplethysmography (OPG) is a simple and widespread method of measuring eye pressure. How often are its results normal in patients with significant bifurcation disease? A number of good reviews in the medical literature deal with the diagnostic accuracy of various OPG methods. OPG permits several categories of carotid occlusive disease to be rated according to the severity of the stenosis. Siekert added that anyone measuring pressures in the eye must interpret the results in the context of the status of the circle of Willis and other intracranial collaterals. Individuals with well-developed collaterals around a carotid obstruction can maintain a good intraocular pressure and give a false normal reading. In addition the OPG, as any other machine, is susceptible to errors in measurement for technical reasons or because of unknown pathological conditions of the eye.

The value of ophthalmodynamometry in evaluating the carotid circulation today was discussed. The opinion of the panel was that the more accurate noninvasive methods available today made ophthalmodynamometry obsolete as a test to detect carotid artery disease.

Young stressed that in patients with ischemic optic neuropathy, OPG measurements do not accomplish the same thing as retinal artery pressure measurements: a patient with temporal arteritis may have normal retinal artery pressures or the latter may be reduced. If the involvement of the central retinal and ciliary arteries is extensive patients may have a reduced OPG reading. In Younge's opinion the fluorescein studies that Hayreh had conducted promised a good way to discriminate between involvement of the central retinal and the ciliary arteries.

ABNORMAL PLATELETS AND RETINAL ISCHEMIA

Gilroy discussed a group of patients with ischemic disease of the retina in whom he had found abnormal platelet aggregation studies. He was asked to comment on the fact that, among the control population, 26% of the individuals also showed platelet abnormalities. He answered that some of the patients in the control group had atherosclerosis, and that of itself may have influenced the behavior of their platelets. He also mentioned that stress will result in abnormal platelet function and speculated that perhaps the fear of a needle puncture to obtain the blood sample might have influenced the result. Clearly much work remains to be done in order to establish platelet abnormality as the etiology of retinal or optic nerve head ischemia. The presence of abnormal platelets in 26% of the controls seems to weaken considerably the cause–effect hypothesis.

Gilroy was asked how far he had pursued the search for carotid disease in these patients with platelet abnormalities. He said he had done prospective ultrasound studies in 20 patients. To the question of whether the platelet abnormalities might be a consequence rather than a cause of arterial occlusion, Gilroy acknowledged that it was a possibility and that he did not have an answer to the question. The problem of what is cause and what is effect with platelet abnormalities goes back to 1963 in Gilroy's experience when he found that patients with acute strokes had abnormal platelets. However, it was not possible to determine whether it was the stroke that caused the platelet abnormality or vice versa. A similar study in patients with TIAs was inconclusive. In his opinion both situations exist: there are platelet abnormalities that may prompt a stroke and there are platelet abnormalities which may be enhanced by a cerebral infarction.

THE QUESTIONS OF "ASYMPTOMATIC" PATIENTS

Traditionally, when arterial pathology is discussed, patients with asymptomatic lesions are presumed to have lesions that are more benign and less threatening than those found in symptomatic patients. In patients with carotid bifurcation disease, for instance, symptomatic lesions are, by general consensus operated upon, while there is controversy as to how to handle asymptomatic but diseased carotids. While there is no doubt that a plaque causing repeated TIAs is generally more virulent than one which produces no symptoms, one cannot assume from the absence of symptoms, the absence of pathological effects. Not uncommonly CT scans show silent frontal or temporal lobe infarcts in patients with presumably "asymptomatic" carotid plaques. Minute digital and plantar skin infarcts are found in patients who have aortic and femoral aneurysms and no symptoms. Once these "silent" manifestations of arterial disease are discovered the patients can no longer be grouped in the same risk category, since their lesions have shown embolic potential, whether clinically obvious or not.

Weiss brought up the fact that, when we analyzed our experience with these patients, we were often puzzled as to how we define an asymptomatic patient. Some of these patients have objective pathology in their eyes of which they are not aware, namely, an embolus in one of the retinal artery branches. As we acquire newer techniques to identify complications of carotid or ophthalmic artery disease (other than those related by the patient) the division of these patients into symptomatic and asymptomatic must be refined. In other words, to presume the innocence of a lesion, the patients must have no signs as well no symptoms.

Magargill elaborated further on the question of asymptomatic patients who have evidence of retinal embolization. He expanded on the relative meaning of the word asymptomatic in these patients. He had seen patients with macular degeneration who did not notice they had a profound loss of vision in one eye until they went in for a pair of glasses. Conversely, there is the case of the artist who can describe and draw the most minute changes in his vision. In his opinion whether patients notice the change in their vision depends very much on how observant they are. Patients may have a total retinal detachment, he said, and walk around for months or even years without knowing that they have a visual impairment.

Clearly, while semantically a patient that does not complain is indeed asymptomatic, uncomplaining patients who have evidence of retinal emboli are obviously a special group that, in terms of risk, would be more properly aligned with those patients who have experienced symptoms.

On the matter of signs and symptoms it was pointed out again that there are patients with no eye complaints in whom one can find a cholesterol plaque in one of the branches of the central retinal artery. There are also patients with absolutely normal ophthalmoscopic findings, who, if they undergo intravenous fluorescence angiography for one reason or another, exhibit tiny branch artery occlusions. Although these patients can in all fairness be called asymptomatic, such findings should put them in a different group altogether.

MANIPULATION OF INTRAOCULAR PRESSURE IN RETINAL ISCHEMIA

Hayreh was asked if in patients with symptoms of retinal ischemia and a low perfusion pressure, he routinely lowers intraocular pressure to increase the perfusion pressure in the eye. He responded that fluorescein angiography is helpful in that a significant delay in ocular perfusion indicates the need to lower the intraocular pressure. He reiterated that perfusion pressure in the eye is equal to mean blood pressure minus intraocular pressure. We seldom increase the mean blood pressure, but we can try to lower intraocular pressure. He related cases where the boxcar patterns of flow in the retinal artery resolved as soon as the intraocular pressure was lowered with drugs. He was adamantly opposed to using paracentesis to lower ocular pressure because in his view it is only a temporary measure, while the use of drugs such as Diamox provides a more lasting decrease in intraocular pressure. Hayreh did not recommend paracentesis in a patient with chronic ischemia; he felt that there was a rebound phenomenon which resulted in the subsequent elevation of intraocular pressure.

The use of retrobulbar anesthetic blocks in patients with acute retinal ischemia was also brought up, and the possibility of causing retrobulbar hemorrhage and blindness with such injections was mentioned. Based on his past experience Hayreh stopped doing retrobulbar injections since he had seen patients get worse, possibly due to the increase in retroocular pressure or perhaps because of a retrobulbar hemorrhage. He did not advise retrobulbar blocks under any circumstances. When questioned about the possibility of increasing intraocular pressure by injection of a certain volume of anesthetic in the retrobulbar space, he did not know how much it would increase intraocular pressure but restated that, without question, one runs the risk of causing a retrobulbar hemorrhage.

“STAINING” OF RETINA AND BLOOD–BRAIN BARRIER

Is the staining of retinal vessels in any way analogous to disruption of the blood–brain barrier? For Magargill the staining of retinal vessels means that the vessels are ischemic because of profound circulatory impairment, and there is breakdown of the blood– retina barrier with leaks also from the iris, the disk, and the whole circulatory system of the eye. He speculated whether these leaks might explain why some of the individuals with this problem think poorly and have poor memory. Their cerebral vessels are also poorly perfused and they may have their blood–brain barrier affected.

ULTRASOUND/ARTERIOGRAPHY

When asked, Higgins stated that all patients with retinal emboli should have ultrasound imaging of the carotids, given that ultrasound can demonstrate small pathological changes which are often missed by arteriograms. (One presumes that if an arteriogram had been done for some reason or other and it were positive, there would be no reason to do ultrasound imaging.) Higgins added that ultrasound imaging may possibly be used to advise arteriographers in which plane there is a greater likelihood of visualizing small carotid irregularities, so the arteriogram does not have to be limited to the traditional anteroposterior and lateral views.

Further discussion of occasional contradictory information given by arteriography and ultrasound imaging, raised the following question: What does one do if the arteriogram is negative and the ultrasound show a lesion? The consensus was that if a patient has transient ischemic attacks, either in the retina or in the cerebral hemispheres and the ultrasound shows a lesion, particularly an ulcerated one which would not be seen in the arteriogram, he or she should have a carotid endarterectomy.

The panel of speakers was also questioned as to what percentage of patients with amaurosis fugax demostrate an embolus on examination of the fundus. The answers ranged from a small to a very small number.

RETINAL VESSELS AND SYSTEMIC BLOOD PRESSURE

In discussing transient retinal symptoms and the possibility of spasm of the retinal arteries, Jampel mentioned that he had seen the retinal arteries go into spasm only once in a woman with eclampsia. The relationship between systemic hypertension and spasm of the retinal arteries was disavowed by Hayreh. He discussed his findings in 60 monkeys in which malignant hypertension was produced by the Goldblatt method. Goldblatt examined the monkeys using fluorescein angiography before and after the creation of hypertension. While many abnormalities were noted in the carotid arteries and in other vascular beds, none were found in the retinal vessels. Hayreh concluded by saying that the estimate of retinal vascular changes in hypertension is exaggerated in clinical medicine.

A question addressed the relationship between narrowed arteries as seen through the ophthalmoscope and perfusion pressure. Hayreh responded that in some patients one may barely touch the eyeball and the central retinal artery starts pulsating (closing). Even these obviously hypotensive arteries have a normal-size lumen. In his opinion, perfusion pressure does not correlate closely with the size of the artery, and that one cannot assess what the perfusion pressure is by looking at the vessel. Concerning the response of the retinal circulation to changes in perfusion pressure, Magargill pointed out that the retinal circulation is auto-regulated and not innervated. Changes in retinal vascular resistance that might have been measured previously with changes in systemic blood pressures may reflect the response of the ophthalmic artery to its sympathetic innervation. Hayreh pointed out that autoregulation operates in a narrow range, and beyond the limits of this range, it ceases to be operative.

The panel observed that the caliber of the retinal arterioles is not a clue to the presence or absence of ocular ischemia unless the flow is so sluggish that acute boxcarting of the blood column can be visualized.

FLUORESCEIN ANGIOGRAPHY IN EYE TIAS

The role of arteriography in patients presenting with transient ocular ischemic attacks generated many questions from the audience. Magargill was asked whether fluorescein angiography would be helpful in such patients even if the appearance of the fundus was normal. Margargill stated that in lesions of the carotid artery which are not hemodynamically significant, the fluorescein timing tends to be normal. However, he stated that when an embolus passes through the retinal circulation and impacts temporarily in it, one can see focal staining in the fluorescein angiogram. A high percentage of patients with such focal staining will have ulcerative lesions in the carotid. Magargil said that, in his experience, 70% of the patients with amaurosis fugax have a carotid lesion. The yield for carotid lesions will be even higher in patients that show staining in the fluorescein angiogram, evidence of impaction and fragmentation of an embolus. These patients in his opinion should have arteriographic studies.

Magargill was asked if, in patients with central retinal artery occlusion, there was any clinical difference between those who had normal choroidal filling on fluorscein angiography and those who had abnormal filling. Magargill found that the worse the visual acuity on presentation, the more likely the patient was to have choroidal as well as retinal circulatory impairment. In other words, the more choroidal involvement, the more the retina is deprived of its secondary circulation and the less likelihood of visual recovery.

CAROTID DISEASE AND ISCHEMIA OF THE EYE

The panel estimated the proportion of patients with carotid artery bifurcation disease that develop symptoms or signs of ischemia of the eye. Young stated that of all patients evaluated at the Mayo Clinic for carotid disease, about 20% of them had eye complaints or some history of visual disturbance. Of the total group, approximately another 20% will have had eye findings such as cholesterol emboli or a substantial difference in retinal artery pressure without eye symptoms. Thus, of the entire group of patients with disease of the carotid bifurcation, 40% will have eye symptoms or abnormal eye findings. The rest of the panel thought that the referral's pattern of their practices would make their answers statistically biased, and they would not be able to draw valid epidemiological conclusions. Thus, they considered themselves unable to estimate the frequency of eye findings (signs or symptoms) in patients with carotid bifurcation disease.

Young's estimates prompted a member of the audience to wonder how it is that vascular surgeons see relatively few patients referred by ophthalmologists when the incidence of signs or symptoms in the eye of 40% among patients with carotid artery disease. Hayreh thought that it was a question of awareness of the link between carotid artery disease and ischemic disease of the eye. In his opinion many ophthalmologists prefer not to treat an otherwise asymptomatic cholesterol embolus so long as the patient does not have any complaints. He sensed that there was considerable reluctance among ophthalmologists to order regular arteriograms in this circumstance, there being a general feeling that this commits the patient to a risky test which may prompt a risky operation.

FLUORESCEIN ANGIOGRAPHY AND GENERAL ANESTHESIA

A member of the audience asked how many opthalmologists were doing fluorescein angiography under general anesthesia. The answer being none, he informed the panel that general anesthesia may be responsible for important variations in the appearance time of the fluorescein dye in the orbital structures. The questioner had experience with fluorescein angiography in children under general endotrachial anesthesia who are intentionally hyperventilated down to a pCO_2 of 28 torr. He stated that the ophthalmic artery behaves like an intracerebral artery: its flow slows down as the vessel constricts with hyperventilation, unlike the external carotid artery which dilates up to a degree. He takes advantage of this fact when he does catheter embolization of external carotid artery branches, hyperventilating his patients to dilate the external carotid territory.

The issue of venous stasis retinopathy-ocular hypoperfusion syndrome generated much debate. Hayreh believes that venous stasis retinopathy is always an outflow or venous problem, and that the so-called ocular hypoperfusion syndrome caused by arterial inflow problems does not exist. Magargill indicated that he found 70% of patients with findings of venous stasis retinopathy had obvious carotid artery disease on digital subtraction arteriography. Magargill pointed out that even though only a small percentage of people with internal carotid artery occlusion develop venous stasis retinopathy, arterial obstruction could still be a cause of this syndrome. Other factors may precipitate the development of venous stasis retinopathy over the long course of carotid artery disease. For instance, the presence of good collaterals from the other side may compensate adequately for awhile and give a normal appearance to the fundus. However when these collaterals cease to be effective as disease develops in the opposite branch, venous stasis may then appear.

III

BETWEEN THE CAROTID AND THE EYE

10

EMBRYOLOGY OF THE ORBITAL AND OCULAR CIRCULATION

David M. Worthen, M.D.

BACKGROUND

Knowledge of the embryology of the arteries and veins of the orbit helps one to understand the adult configuration. An anatomic characteristic of arteries in the adult is that, within the eye, they form three cones. The first lies centrally, within the apex where arteries come forward to supply the globe itself. The middle cone of vessels supplies muscular branches and the peripheral cone of arterial branches supplies the orbital rim. These three systems of vessels—central, middle, and peripheral— are in contrast to the veins that tend to lie on the periphery of the muscle cone and are tightly encased in a series of connective tissue septa which also give support to the globe (1). This description of the adult orbit has appeared in a series of articles by Drs. Koornneef (2) and Bergen (3) at the University of Amsterdam. Their findings are based upon a meticulous analysis of celloidin-embedded, 60 micron, serial sections from a series of adult human orbits. Dr. Bergen's review of the literature on the vascular system of the human orbit is a milestone summary of the literature and includes the major review articles (4). The 90 references listed by Dr. Bergen will easily provide the ambitious reader with a review of the last 100 years of work defining the normal anatomy of the human orbit and eye. They include the landmark publications by Whitnal, Sudakevitch, and Hayreh.

The contemporary summary of the anatomy and embryology of the arteries in the human orbit was most adequately presented by Dr. Sohan Singh Hayreh when he was the Beit Memorial Reseach Fellow with the Institute of Ophthalmology at the University of London and was honored by being able to present the Arris and Gale Lecture at the Royal College of Surgeons of England in May 1963. That presentation was published in the

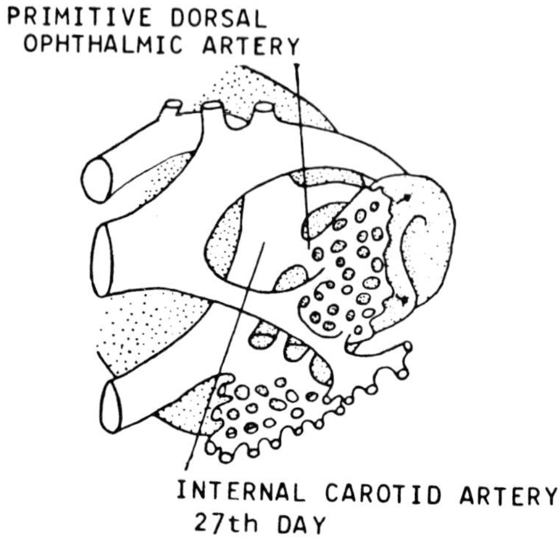

Fig. 10.1. In 27-day-old embryo, internal carotid artery gives rise to primitive dorsal ophthalmic artery. (Reproduced with permission of the American Academy of Ophthalmology from the self-instruction manual by Anthony A. Pearson, Ph.D., 1975.)

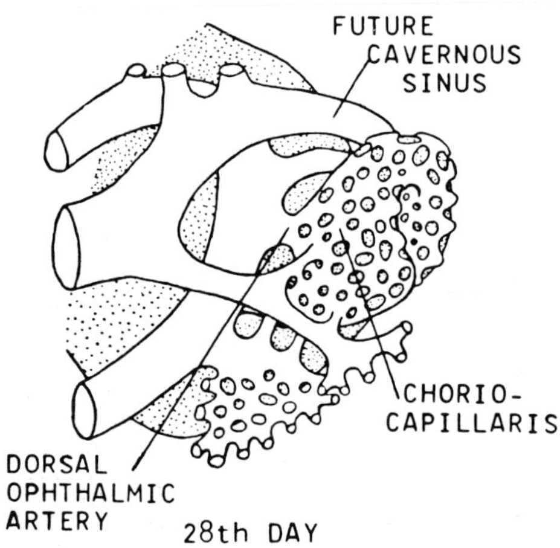

Fig. 10.2. By day 28, future choriocapillaris is wrapping around optic cup and future cavernous sinus venous drainage system is forming. (Reproduced with permission of the American Academy of Ophthalmology from the self-instruction manual by Anthony A. Pearson, Ph.D., 1975.)

British Journal of Surgery in that same year (5). Little has been added to the literature on embryology since this summary, which includes some 92 references.

A visual summary of the embryology of the orbit can be obtained by viewing the American Academy of Ophthalmology's videotape taken from the original one-hour film prepared by the late Dr. George Smetzler and available from the Academy for either rent or purchase.

Anatomical Description

During the involution of the first two aortic arches, the primitive carotid artery emerges and divides into two main branches near the top of the optic vesicle. Inferiorly, that division forms the posterior communicating artery. The superior or cranial portion turns anterior and ventral to go around the

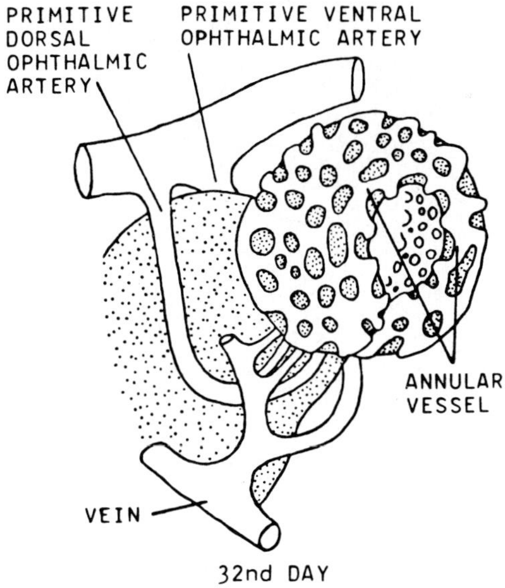

Fig. 10.3. By day 32, annular vessels are formed around opening in optic cup and both primitive dorsal and ventral ophthalmic arteries are differentiated. (Reproduced with permission of the American Academy of Opthalmology from the self-instruction manual by Anthony A. Pearson, Ph.D., 1975.)

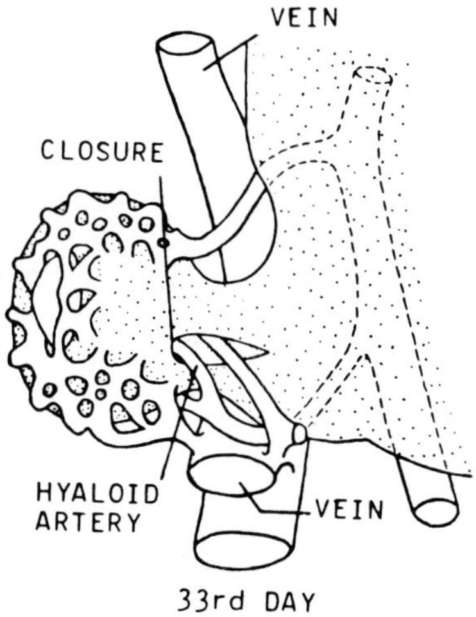

Fig. 10.4. By day 33, the hyaloid artery arising from the primitive dorsal ophthalmic artery is trapped by the closing of the fetal cleft. (Reproduced with permission of the American Academy of Opthalmology from the self-instruction manual by Anthony A. Pearson, Ph.D., 1975.)

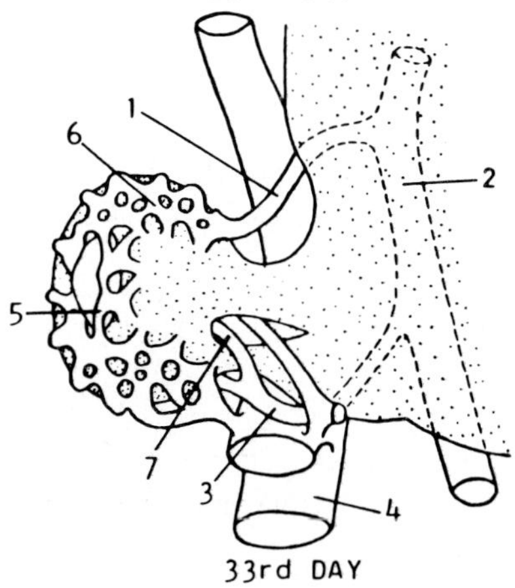

Fig. 10.5. The structures seen on the 33rd day are: 1, primitive ventral ophthalmic artery; 2, internal carotid artery; 3, primitive dorsal ophthalmic artery; 4, cavernous sinus; 5, annular vessels; 6, choriocapillaris; and 7, hyaloid artery.(Reproduced with permission of the American Academy of Opthalmology from the self-instruction manual __________, by Anthony A. Pearson, Ph.D., 1975.)

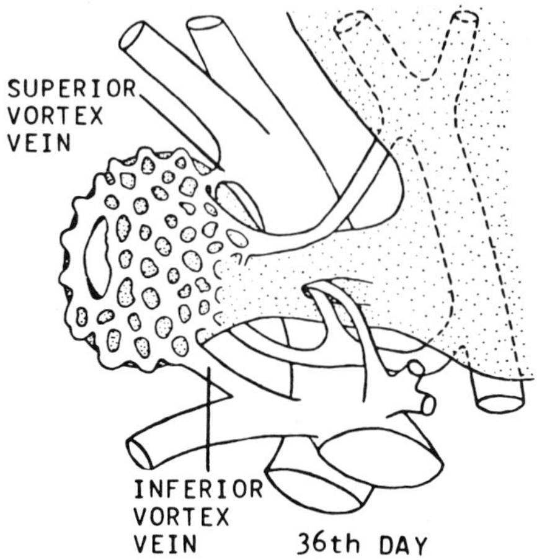

Fig. 10.6. By 36th day, superior and inferior vortex veins are well developed and future internal circulation of eye is defined with hyaloid artery and future retinal vein emerging from closing fetal cleft. (Reproduced with permission of the American Academy of Opthalmology from the self-instruction manual by Anthony A. Pearson, Ph.D., 1975.)

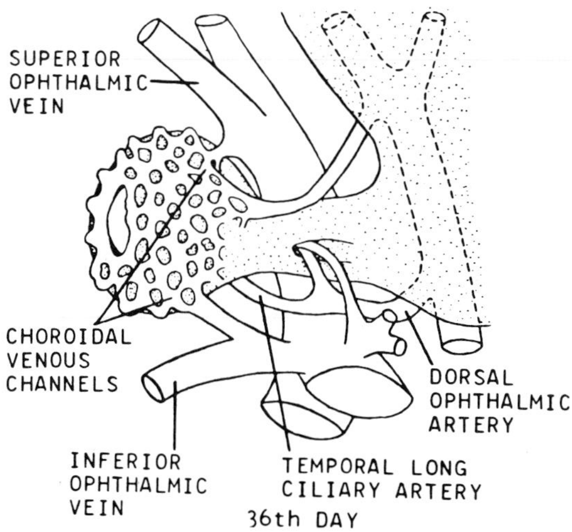

Fig. 10.7. By 36th day, superior and inferior ophthalmic vein and continuation of dorsal ophthalmic artery into orbit show future sites of adult configuration with central arterial cone and peripheral venous drainage encased within fascia of orbit. (Reproduced with permission of the American Academy of Opthalmology from the self-instruction manual by Anthony A. Pearson, Ph.D., 1975.)

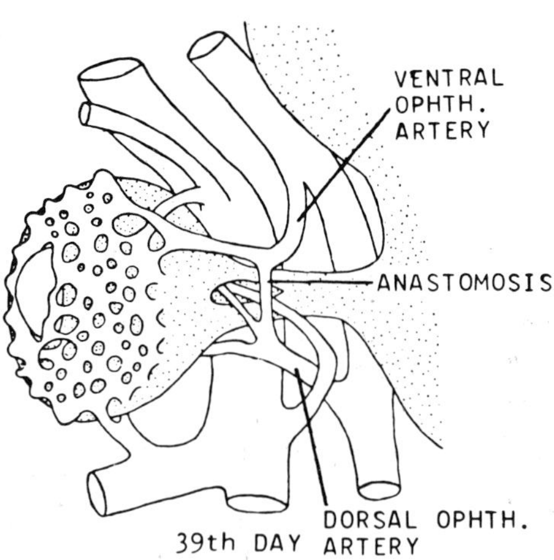

Fig. 10.8. Anastomosis between ventral and dorsal ophthalmic artery on 39th day may contribute to vascular ring around optic nerve discussed in text. (Reproduced with permission of the American Academy of Opthalmology from the self-instruction manual by Anthony A. Pearson, Ph.D., 1975.)

base of the optic vesicle. It is this cranial division from which several collateral branches arise. Those branches are the anterior carotid artery, the middle cerebral artery, and the anterior cerebral artery. At the terminal end of the anterior cerebral artery is a primitive olfactory artery.

In his review, Hayreh gives credit to the 1948 publication by Padget on the development of the human ophthalmic artery. Padget recounts that the formation of the definitive arterial system is from a very diffuse plexus of capillaries that gradually leads to the disappearance of certain vessels and the hypertrophy of others.

What will eventually be known as the ophthalmic artery has a rather complicated evolution and arises late in development. On approximately the 27th day, several small vessels appear in the mesoderm around the optic vesicle leading from the internal carotid artery and extending a short distance forward (Figure 10.1). Most of the primitive eye is supplied by this branch of the internal carotid artery which arises near where it bifurcates on the side opposite the posterior communicating artery. It is given the term the primitive dorsal ophthalmic artery. Its position is inferior and dorsal to the optic cup and the stalk and supplies both of them.

The venous plexus into which this primitive dorsal ophthalmic artery drains can be seen by the 28th day and will eventually become the cavernous sinus system (Figure 10.2). When the branches of the primitive dorsal ophthalmic artery have developed forward to the front of the optic cup, some of them turn inward hugging the fundus, while others anastomose along the rim to form the annular vessels (Figure 10.3).

A second vessel, the primitive ventral ophthalmic artery, arises from the internal carotid artery behind the stalk and leads to the ventral, cranial, and medial part of the plexus around the optic vesicle (Figure 10.4). The primitive dorsal ophthalmic artery gives rise to the hyaloid artery going through the fetal cleft and forward to the lens (Figure 10.5). As the fissure closes, this network of vessels inside the cup is trapped except for a small branch which connects the ophthalmic artery through the opening in the stalk behind the cup. That branch is the hyaloid artery and goes forward to form a tunic around the lens. In addition to forming this vascular network, it also contributes to the formation of the primary vitreous (Figure 10.6).

At this stage, veins begin to appear in the optic nerve and parallel the hyaloid artery. The inferior and superior vortex veins are apparent by the 36th day (Figure 10.7). The original artery distal to the hyaloid artery forms a common temporal ciliary artery or lateral posterior ciliary artery.

Therefore, the permanent ophthalmic artery represents the primitive dorsal ophthalmic artery and reaches its adult position after considerable caudal migration of the primitive dorsal ophthalmic artery along the choroid artery (Figure 10.8). The original primitive dorsal ophthalmic

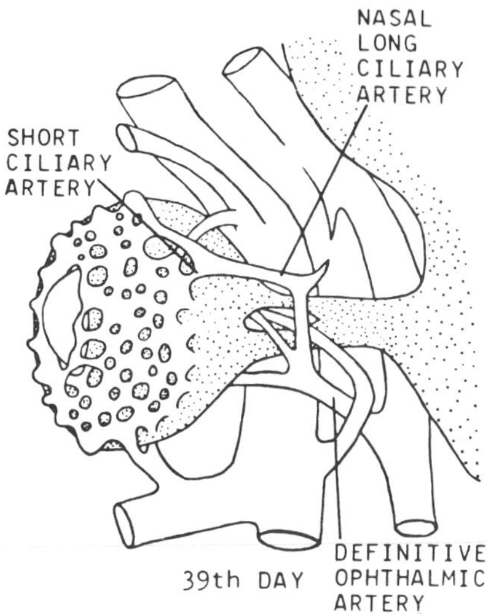

Fig. 10.9. Ventral ophthalmic artery forms nasal long ciliary artery. Dorsal ophthalmic artery will be definitive ophthalmic artery and give rise to temporal long ciliary artery. (Reproduced with permission of the American Academy of Opthalmology from the self-instruction manual by Anthony A. Pearson, Ph.D., 1975.)

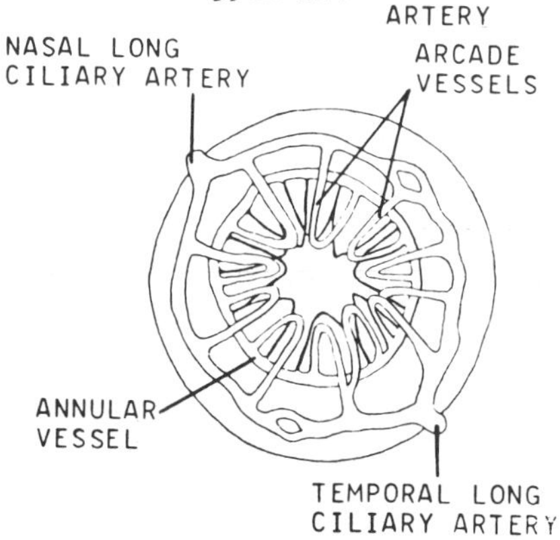

Fig. 10.10. Two long ciliary arteries contribute to annular vessels which branch into arcade vessels forming pupillary membrane of iris. (Reproduced with permission of the American Academy of Opthalmology from the self-instruction manual by Anthony A. Pearson, Ph.D., 1975.)

artery was quite cranial or anterior to the optic stock, but in the adult position, it moves to a posterior or caudal position with reference to the stalk. This migration takes place by means of a series of anastomotic loops as the expanding brain and cerebral arteries become more withdrawn from the developing optic nerve and the eye itself.

Development of the orbital roof and the future optic foramen completes this process and relegates the ophthalmic artery to a permanent origin below the level of the carotid siphon.

Venous channels differentiate in the mesoderm adjacent to the pigment layer of the cup, and through it blood is drained into an upper and a lower venous plexis and hence, into what is to become the cavernous sinus (see figure 10.7). In the meantime, the ventral ophthalmic artery has anastomosed with the definitive ophthalmic and the distal portion will become the nasal long ciliary or medial posterior ciliary artery (Figure 10.9). This anastomosis takes place ventral to the optic nerve and is usually linked with the hyaloid branch of the ophthalmic artery. At this point, there is an interruption of the primitive ventral ophthalmic artery proximal to the second anastomosis so that the posterior ciliary artery on the medial aspect arises in common with that of the origin of the central retinal artery (Figure 10.10).

By the 40th day of the embryo, all of the ocular branches of the ophthalmic artery have been established. The ophthalmic artery is the only branch from the internal carotid artery to the eye. Meanwhile, the venous system has further developed and forms both the vortex and ophthalmic veins. Within the eye, the anterior chamber is starting to appear and the pupillary membrane behind it is being fed by arterial loops and arcades sprouting from the annular vessels. These sprouting arcade vessels will eventually form the anterior surface of the iris and when they atrophy, will leave a collarette that can be seen at the slitlamp. As more circulation occurs in the anterior system, there is a gradual atrophy of vessels in the primary vitreous leaving an area identified in the adult as Cloquet's canal. In the choroid, the layer of large venous channels will drain directly to the vortex vein and towards the end of the fourth month, two arteries sprouting from the hyaloid artery will begin the vascularization of the retina.

Another contribution to the orbit begins when the second pharyngeal artery gives origin to the stapedial artery on approximately the 39th day. This has two primary divisions. One accompanies the ophthalmic division of the trigeminal nerve anteriorly and is called the supraorbital branch. The other accompanies the maxillary and mandibular divisions of the fifth nerve and forms the counterpart arterial system. By the 40th day, the supraorbital branch enters the orbit. By the 42nd day, the ophthalmic artery stem anastomoses with the supraorbital division of the stapedial artery. At a later stage, the stapedial artery will lose its connection with the second arch artery and through its maxillo-mandibular division become annexed by the maxillary division of the external carotid. It is this joining of the maxillo-mandibular and the supraorbital divisions of the stapedial artery which forms the ultimate middle meningeal artery.

In Hayreh's study of 170 orbital specimens, he found the origin of the blood supply to the eye was from this middle meningeal artery in six cases. In four cases, he saw partial blood supply from the middle meningeal artery with a big trunk arising from the middle meningeal and a small one from the internal carotid artery.

All of the orbital branches of the adult ophthalmic artery are derived from the supraorbital division of the stapedial artery. By the 45th day, three branches arise from that division; the frontal, the supraorbital, and anterior ethmoid. After the 45th day, the stem of the lacrimal artery develops.

By the 45th day, the optic nerve at the origin of these three primary ocular branches of the ophthalmic artery is surrounded by an arterial ring, the components of which represent a number of secondary anastamoses. The less well developed central portion represents the anastomosis between the primitive ventral ophthalmic artery and the ophthalmic stem. The dorsal part of the ring is longer and probably of more recent origin and is responsible for the definitive ophthalmic artery arising from the ventral to the dorsal aspect of the nerve. A small ventral portion of this ring usually disappears while the other parts are retained leading to one of the two configurations of the adult ophthalmic artery.

Padget postulated and Hayreh confirmed in 59 specimens that in the majority of cases there was a loss of the connection between the supraorbital branch of the stapedial and the primitive ventral ophthalmic artery. Next most common was a break between the primitive ventral and dorsal arteries, then a break between the supraorbital and stapedial, and least often, atrophy of the segment of the supraorbital branch of the stapedial artery between the latter two. The origin of the muscular branches varies, depending upon which of these portions of the embryonic ring disappear. When the ophthalmic artery crosses under the optic nerve, the medial muscular branches are usually independent branches arising after or at the same place as the medial posterior ciliary artery from the second part of the ophthalmic artery.

Therefore, the crossing of the ophthalmic artery either over or under the optic nerve depends upon which segment of the ring has disappeared. In Hayreh's series, 83% of the time the artery passed over the nerve and in 17% it passed underneath the nerve.

This brief review of the embryology of the vascular system of the eye and orbit should help to put in context the variation in both arterial and venous anatomy noted by arteriography or venography in various conditions of the carotid artery.

REFERENCES

1. Bergen, M.P.: A spatial reconstruction of the orbital vascular pattern in relation with the connective tissue system. *Acta Morphol Neerl Scand* 20:117, 1982.
2. Koornneef, L.: The architecture of the musculufibrous apparatus in the human orbit. *Acta Morphol Neerl Scand* 15:35, 1977.
3. Bergen, M.P.: Relationship between the arteries and veins and connective tissue system in the human orbit I. The retro orbital part of the orbit: apical region. II. Septal complex region (1982b); and III. The bulbar part of the orbit (1982c). *Acta Morphol Neerl Scand.* 20
4. Bergen, M.P.: A literature review of the vascular system in the human orbit. *Acta Morphol Neerl Scand* 19:273, 1981.
5. Hayreh, S.S.: Arteries of the orbit in the human being. *Brit Surg* 50:938, 1963.

11

ANGIOGRAPHIC EVALUATION OF ORBITAL VESSELS

Anton N. Hasso, M.D.

The arterial vascularization of the orbit includes the ophthalmic artery and its branches, along with several important vessels originating from the external carotid artery. The complete angiographic study of the orbit requires both internal and external carotid angiograms.

TECHNIQUE

Serial direct magnification orbital angiography is routinely performed at our institution with an x-ray tube having a 0.1-mm nominal focal spot (1–3). In the anteroposterior projection, the central ray is angled cranially 5–10 degrees to the orbitomeatal line, using a tube–film distance of 90 cm and a tube–object distance of approximately 30 cm for a calculated linear magnification factor of 3.0. Lateral views are obtained with a tube–film distance of 120 cm and a tube–object distance of approximately 45 cm, resulting in a calculated linear magnification factor of 2.67. Subtraction is carried out in all cases and is considered essential in orbital angiography.

The "washout" of the vessels traversing the anterior orbit in the lateral projection, due to the superimposition of the air filled paranasal sinuses, is partially handled by using a specially designed brass wedge filter. The wedge filter is used to absorb a portion of the excess radiation with resultant equalized film exposure. We prefer slightly darker film exposures to adequately penetrate the dense sphenoid and zygomatic bones in order to enhance the subtraction views. Patients are requested to close their eyes during the angiographic series to further facilitate motionless films.

Selective internal and external carotid artery catheterization is customarily accomplished by means of the percutaneous transfemoral ap-

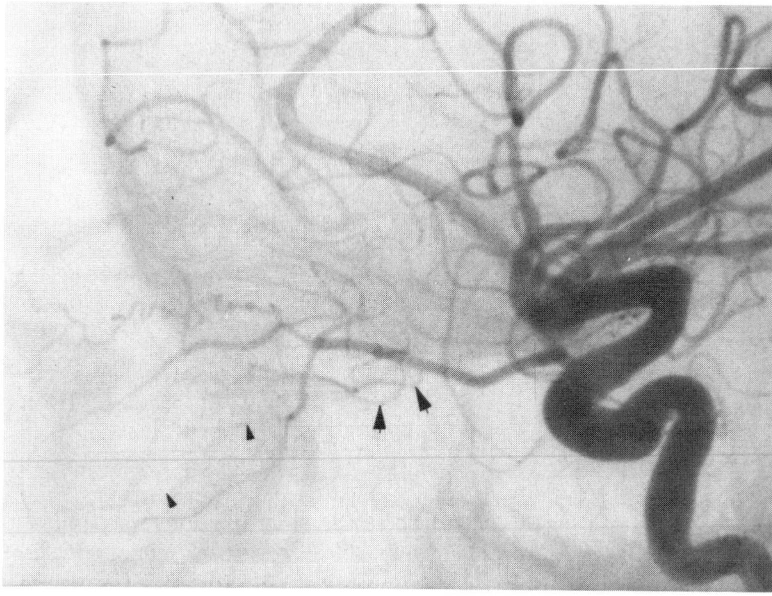

Fig. 11.1. Ophthalmic artery medial to optic nerve. Note the separate origin of two posterior ciliary arteries (*large arrowheads*). The anterior ciliary branches (*small arrowheads*) originate from the inferior medial musclar artery and show a course similar to the rectus muscles.

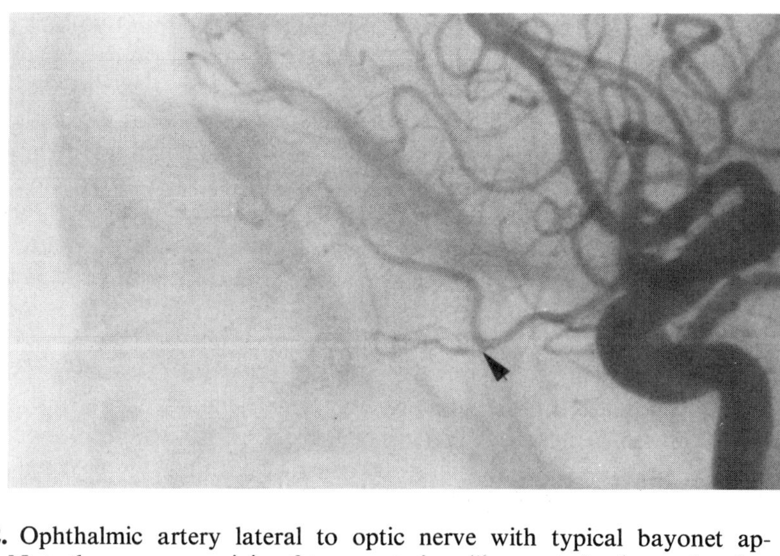

Fig. 11.2. Ophthalmic artery lateral to optic nerve with typical bayonet appearance. Note the common origin of two posterior ciliary arteries (*arrowhead*).

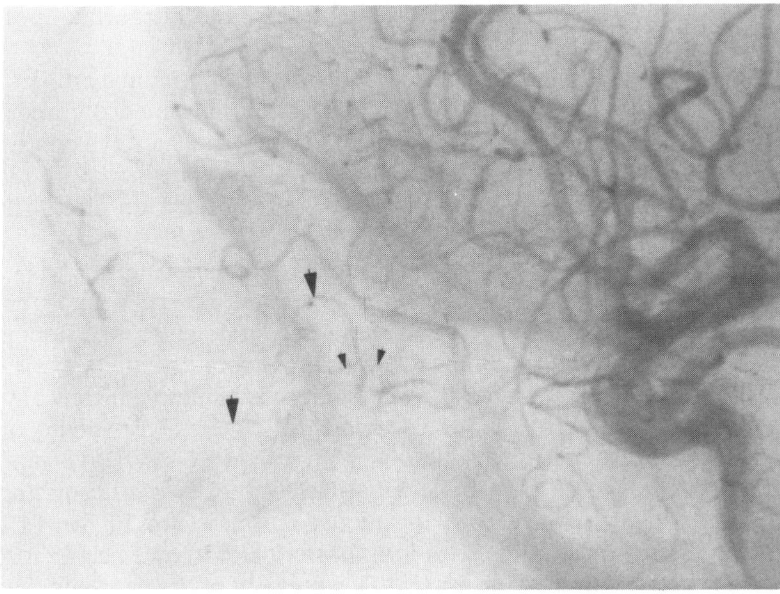

Fig. 11.3. Later phase of Figure 11.2. The short posterior ciliary (*small arrowheads*) and long posterior ciliary arteries (*large arrowheads*) are identified.

proach. The dual blood supply to the orbit is studied separately with complete outline of the anastomotic pathways. However, in cases of carotid bifurcation occlusive disease, only common carotid injections are performed.

OPHTHALMIC ARTERY

The ophthalmic artery, after turning around the optic nerve from inferior to superior, extends anteriorly in a medial direction terminating in the angular and frontal branches (3–6). Just before terminating into these angular and frontal branches, it gives off medial palpebral branches. The first intraorbital branch of the ophthalmic artery is the central retinal artery. A major early branch is the lacrimal artery, extending anteriorly in a superolateral direction. The other major branch is the supraorbital artery which extends between the lacrimal and terminal ophthalmic arteries, but in a higher plane within the orbit. There are several muscular branches to the adenexal structures, ethmoidal branches to the adjacent mucosa, and ciliary branches to the ocular choroid. Several fine intracanalicular collateral vessels are present for the optic nerve, and they form a ring of vessels around the intracranial, intracanalicular, and intraorbital portions of the optic nerve.

There are two basic types of branching of the ophthalmic artery (7). In type A, the ophthalmic artery branches after curving medially about the optic nerve in 17% of cases (Figure 11.1). Type B is where the ophthalmic artery branches after curving laterally about the optic nerve in 73% of cases. Type B gives the classic "bayonet" appearance on lateral angiographic views (Figure 11.2).

The orbital branches of the ophthalmic system are routinely visualized on magnification arteriograms (2). The central retinal artery remains hidden on most angiograms, even with magnification. This is disappointing since its diameter (about 0.3mm) is within the theoretical limits of visibility (4). The posterior ciliary arteries are usually visible angiographically and show a sinusoidal course with one or two short curves before giving off the long and short posterior ciliary branches (Figures 11.1–11.3). The anterior ciliary branches come off of the muscular branches of the ophthalmic artery and travel forward with the rectus muscles (See Figure 11.1) to perforate the sclera and join with long posterior ciliary vessels in forming the major arterial circle of the iris (8). The intensity of the choroidal blush is proportional to the quality of opacification of the ciliary branches.

EXTERNAL CAROTID ARTERY

The blood supply from the external carotid artery to the orbit may be divided into two groups: a superficial periorbital group consisting of the facial, infraorbital, and superficial temporal arteries and an orbito-palpebral group consisting of the middle meningeal, anterior deep temporal, and infraorbital arteries which provide deep anastomoses and contribute significantly to flow in the ophthalmic system (1).

Of interest, is technique-dependent bidirectional flow in certain segments of the orbital anastomotic pathways. Complete orbital angiographic opacification may be accomplished by selective external carotid or subselective maxillary artery angiograms. The understanding of this phenomenon requires a brief review of the embryologic development of the orbital vessels.

Embryology

At the 12–14 mm embryonic stage, the primitive ophthalmic artery develops three terminal branches. The hyaloid branch forms the central retinal artery; the common temporociliary branch forms the lateral ciliary arteries; and the common nasociliary branch forms the medial ciliary

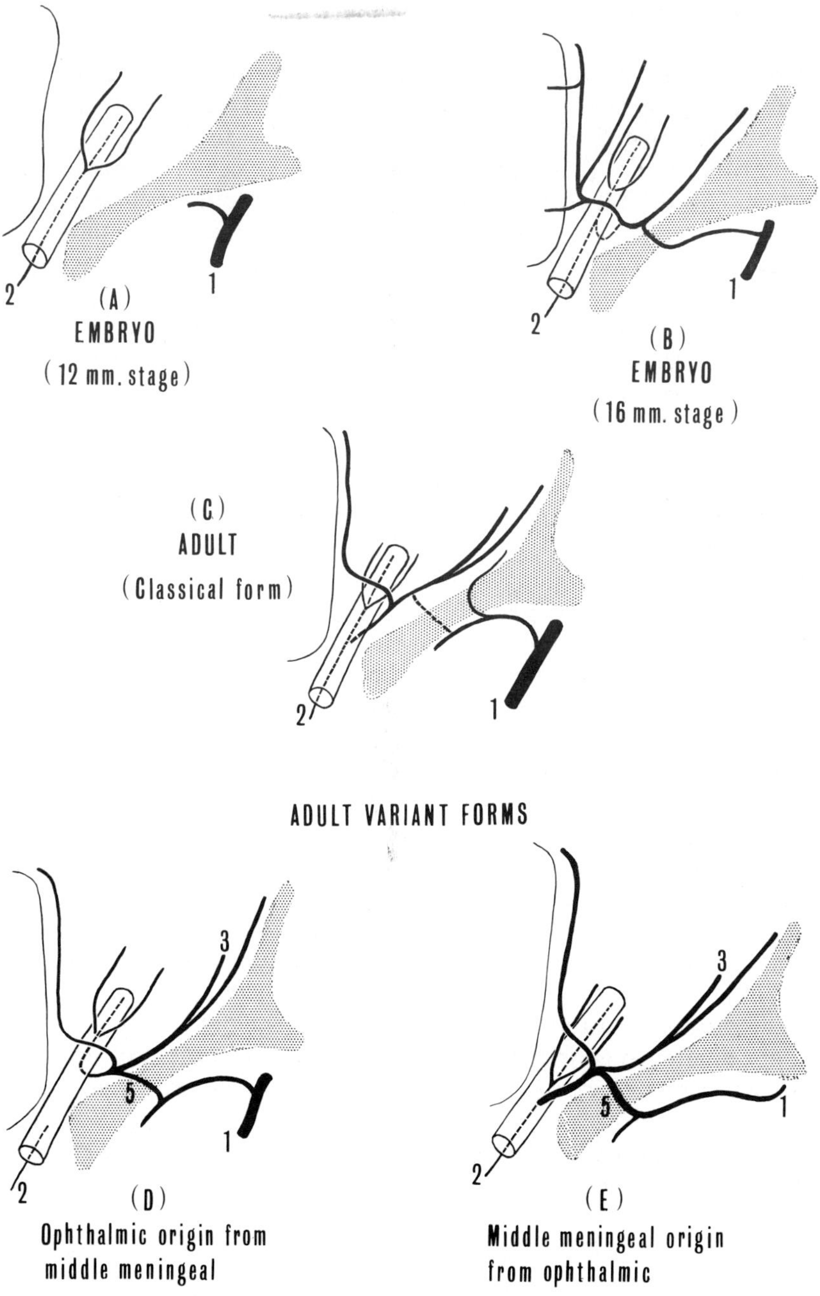

Fig. 11.4. Embryonic development of the orbital vessels. **A:** Embryo (12-mm stage). **B:** Embryo (16-mm stage). **C:** Adult (classic form). **D:** Adult variant form (ophthalmic origin from middle meningeal). **E:** Adult variant form (middle meningeal origin from ophthalmic).

arteries. This primitive system consists only of neurosensory branches and depends fully on the internal carotid artery (Figure 11.4A) (1, 2).

At the 14–16 mm embryonic stage, the orbital branch of the supraorbital artery (stapedial artery) becomes annexed to the ophthalmic system. This orbital artery branches into the ethmoidonasal artery (which will later give rise to the third portion of the definitive ophthalmic artery), the frontal artery (which will give rise to the adult supraorbital artery), and the lacrimal artery (which remains as the adult lacrimal artery). An anastomosis between the orbital system and the primitive ophthalmic system occurs and later forms the second portion of the definitive ophthalmic artery (Figure 11.4B).

After partial regression of the proximal portion of the orbital artery occurs, it is called the recurrent meningeal artery. The stapedial artery will become the adult maxillary artery after its annexation by the external carotid artery. Later, the supraorbital artery forms the middle meningeal artery (Figure 11.4C).

The recurrent meningeal artery is an adult remnant of a common meningoorbital vascular embryonic system. The recurrent meningeal artery anastomoses the lacrimal artery with the anterior branch of the middle meningeal artery in the lateral-most portion of the superior orbital fissure. This vessel may be abnormally developed in three situations:

(a) If the proximal ophthalmic artery regresses and the embryonic orbital artery persists, the adult ophthalmic artery then "originates" form the middle meningeal artery (Figure 11.4D).

(b) If the embryonic supraorbital artery regresses and the embryonic orbital artery persists, the middle meningeal artery "originates" from the ophthalmic artery (Figure 11.4E).

(c) If the embryonic orbital-ophthalmic anastomosis does not take place, then the orbit is supplied by two trunks: one issued from the internal carotid artery for the optic nerve and retina; the other issued from the middle meningeal artery to supply the rest of the orbit.

The meningolacrimal artery originates from the anterior branch of the middle meningeal artery, similar to the origin of the recurrent meningeal artery. The territory supplied by this vessel depends on the development of the lacrimal branch of the ophthalmic artery. The lateral portion of the orbit or lacrimal territory is supplied by either or both of these vessels (Figure 11.5).

EXTERNAL CAROTID TO OPHTHALMIC COLLATERALS

Cases of internal carotid occlusion show a network of collaterals from the external carotid artery to the ophthalmic artery (1). The facial artery

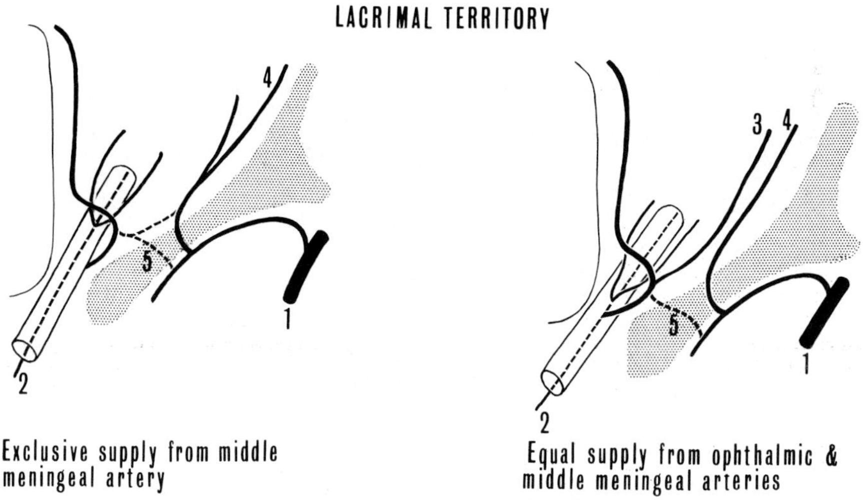

Fig. 11.5. Blood supply to the lacrimal territory. **A:** Exclusive supply from middle meningeal artery. **B:** Equal supply from ophthalmic and middle meningeal arteries. Key for Figures 11.4, 11.5: 1, Stapedial artery; 2, ophthalmic artery with its branches; 3, lacrimal artery; 4, meningolacrimal artery; 5, recurrent meningeal artery.

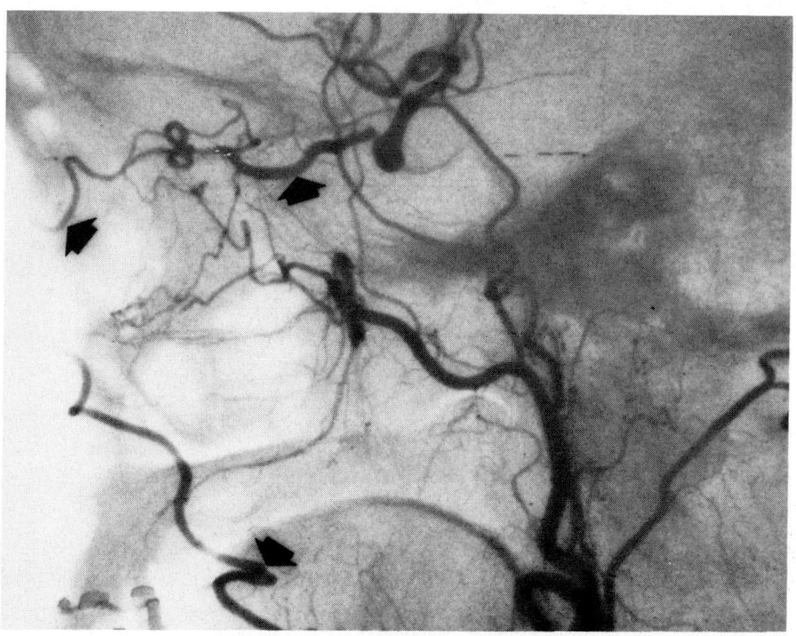

Fig. 11.6. Internal carotid artery occlusion. Note the retrograde collateral filling of the angular branch of the ophthalmic artery from the facial branch of the external carotid artery (*arrowheads*).

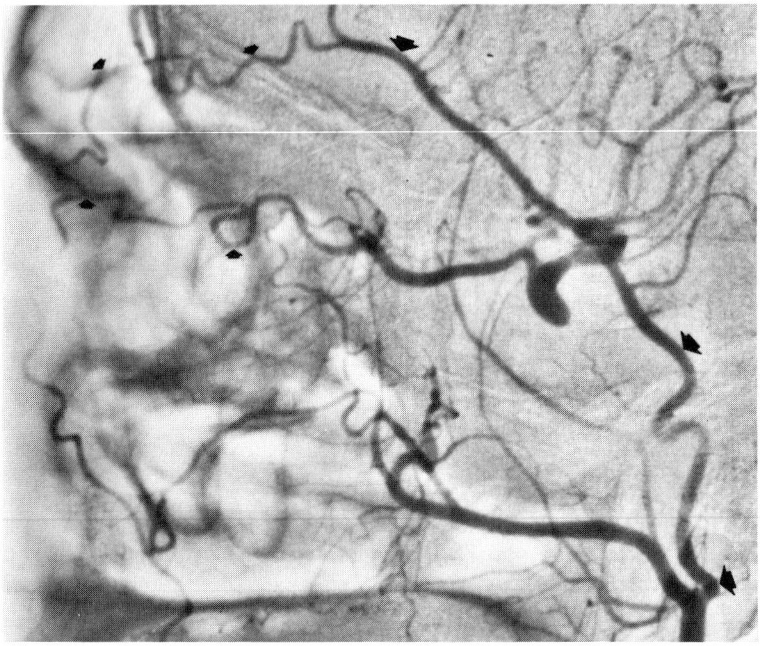

Fig. 11.7. Internal carotid artery occlusion. Note the flow from the superficial temporal artery (*large arrowheads*) to the ophthalmic artery (*small arrowheads*) via the frontal branch.

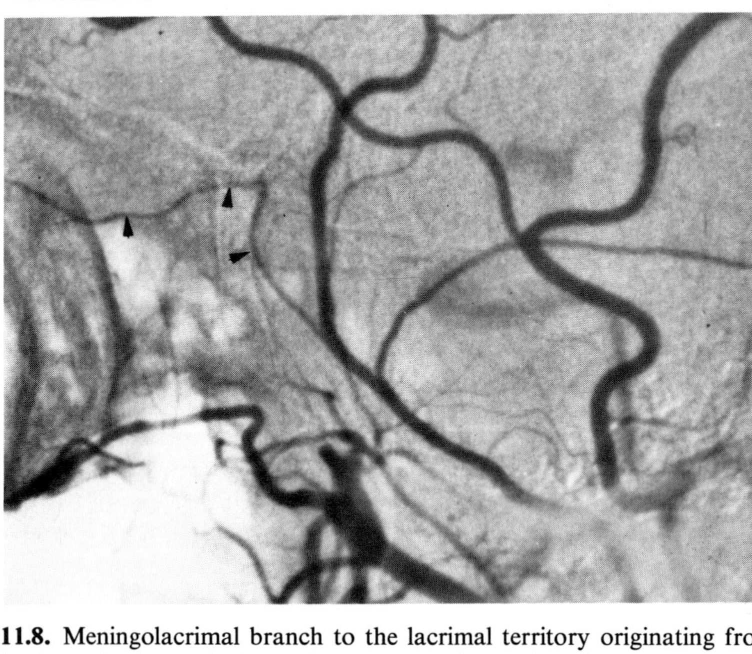

Fig. 11.8. Meningolacrimal branch to the lacrimal territory originating from the anterior branch of the middle meningeal artery (*arrowheads*).

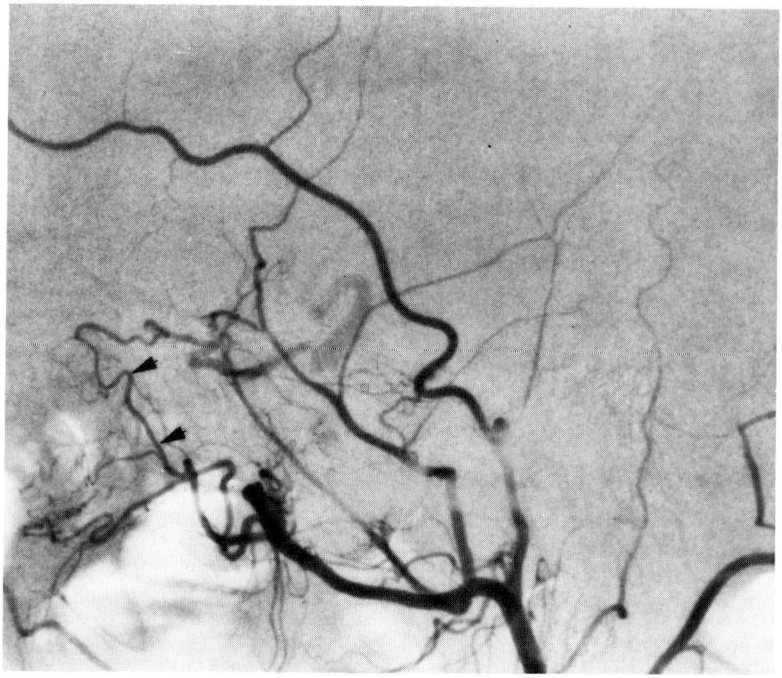

Fig. 11.9. Internal carotid artery occlusion. Note the lacrimal branch of the anterior deep temporal artery (*arrowheads*) anastomosing with the lacrimal branch of the ophthalmic artery.

anastomoses directly to the terminal angular branch of the ophthalmic artery (Figure 11.6). Superficial collaterals to the palpebral ophthalmic branches originate from the infraorbital artery after it exits the infraorbital canal below the orbit. The superficial temporal artery has normal physiologic connections to the supraorbital and terminal frontal branches of the ophthalmic artery (Figure 11.7). There also are zygomaticomalar and transverse facial to palpebral collaterals from the superficial temporal artery.

The blood supply to the orbit from the middle meningeal artery was discussed above in the embryology section. The lacrimal territory is supplied by the meningolacrimal artery in 30% of cases (Figure 11.8) and consists of three regions: an upper one for the lacrimal gland, a middle one for the lacrimal gland and eyelid, and a lower one for the muscles. The inferior territory has collateral branches from the infraorbital and anterior deep temporal arteries.

The orbital branches of the anterior deep temporal artery supply the lateral lacrimal territory entering the orbit through the inferior orbital fissure (Figure 11.9) or directly through the zygomatic bone. The deep portion of the infraorbital artery gives rise to several other orbital branches that enter the orbit through the inferior orbital fissure which joins the muscular ophthalmic branches.

CONCLUSIONS

It is evident that both the ophthalmic artery and the external carotid artery are responsible for orbital blood supply, resulting in a large number of collateral channels between them. A thorough understanding of orbital arteriography is aided by a knowledge of the external carotid artery contibutions to orbital vascularization.

REFERENCES

1. Lasjaunias, P., Vignaud, J. and Hasso, A.N.: Maxillary artery blood supply to the orbit: normal and pathological aspects. *Neuroradiology* 9:87, 1975.
2. Vignaud, J., Hasso, A.N., Lasjaunias, P. and Clay, C.: Orbital vascular anatomy and embryology. *Radiology* 111:617, 1974.
3. Wolfe, E.: The vessels. In: *The Anatomy of the Eye and Orbit.* 4th ed. New York: McGraw-Hill, pp. 426–479.
4. Di Chiro, G.: Ophthalmic arteriography. *Radiology* 77:948, 1961.
5. Duke-Elder, S.S., and Cook, C.: Ocular vascular systems. In: Duke-Elder, S.S., ed. *System of Ophthalmology.* vol. 3. St. Louis: C.V. Mosby, 1961, pp. 179–208.
6. Duke-Elder, S.S., and Wybar, K.C.: Orbital vascular system. In: Duke-Elder, S.S., ed. *System of Ophthalmology.* vol. 2. St. Louis: C.V. Mosby, pp. 246–270.
7. Vignaud, J., Clay, C., and Aubin, M.L.: Orbital arteriography. *Radiol. Clin. North Am.* 10:39, 1972.
8. Torczynski, E.: Choroid and suprachoroid. In: Jakobiec, F.A., ed. *Ocular Anatomy, Embryology, and Teratology.* Philadelphia: Harper and Row, 1982, pp. 553–585.
9. Wende, S. and Schindler, K.: Technique and use of x-ray magnification in cerebral arteriography. *Neuroradiology* 1:117, 1970.

12

POSTERIOR CILIARY ARTERIES: Their Anatomy, Distribution and Occlusive Disorders

Sohan Singh Hayreh, M.D., Ph.D

Extensive anatomical studies of the choroidal vascular bed have been conducted, mostly by studying casts prepared by postmortem injection of a variety of materials and recently by using scanning electron microscopy to study casts. These studies have formed the basis of the classical anatomical textbook description of the choroidal vasculature. According to most of these descriptions, (a) Extensive anastomoses exist between the various branches of all the short posterior ciliary arteries (PCAs), so that occlusion of one vessel ordinarily should not produce infarction of the choroid; (b) the short PCAs anastomose with the anterior ciliary arteries at the equator of the eye; and (c) the choriocapillaris is arranged in one plane as a single continuous layer of wide lumen capillaries and they form a continuous anastomotic network over the entire choroid.

However, it is well known that inflammatory, metastatic, ischemic and degenerative lesions in the choroid are usually localized. Moreover, a number of clinical and experimental observations reported in the literature suggest that the PCAs have a segmental supply to the choroid. In view of these conflicting observations and with the advent of fluorescein angiography, which has enabled us to study not only the blood flow but also the physiological anatomy in vivo, we and a number of other workers have investigated the choroidal vascular bed in vivo. These studies have almost revolutionized our concept of the choroidal vascular bed and helped to explain the pathogenesis of some obscure fundus lesions.

ANATOMY OF THE POSTERIOR CILIARY ARTERIES

There is a good deal of confusion as to the nomenclature, number, origin, and distribution of the PCAs in man. I have described the subject in detail elsewhere (1).

Number: The ophthalmic artery in humans gives out one (in 3%), two (in 48%), three (in 39%), four (in 8%), or five (in 2%) PCAs. When there are more than three PCAs, the additional arteries are usually small in size.

Nomenclature: I have designated the PCAs according to their relation to the optic nerve near their site of entry into the eyeball. They are called:

(a) *Medial PCA:* This lies medial to the optic nerve and may be one (in about 70%) or two (in about 30%) in number.

(b) *Lateral PCA:* This lies lateral to the optic nerve, and there may be one (in about 75%), two (in about 20%), three (in about 3%), or none (in about 3%) in number.

(c) *Superior PCA:* This is seen in only 9% of the total population and may be one (in 7%) or two (in 2%) in number; these are usually small in size.

The various PCAs run forward, divide into a large number of small branches and pierce the sclera near the optic nerve. Out of these branches of the PCAs, one on the medial and another one on the lateral side, form the long PCAs, while the rest are called the short PCAs. The number of short PCAs piercing the sclera varies from about 10 to 20, depending upon the number of times the PCAs have subdivided before reaching the sclera. From this account it is evident that there are three types of PCAs:

(a) *Main PCAs:* These arise from the ophthalmic artery and are usually 2 to 3 (usually medial and lateral PCAs).

(b) *Long PCAs:* These are 2 in number, one medial and the other lateral.

(c) *Short PCAs:* These may be 10 to 20.

I want to stress very strongly that unless this terminology is clearly understood and adhered to, there may be tremendous confusion.

PHYSIOLOGICAL ANATOMY OF THE CHOROIDAL VASCULAR BED

In vivo clinical and experimental fluorescein fundus angiographic studies have clearly demonstrated that the choroidal blood flow is segmental, almost like that seen in the retinal vasculature. The findings are described in detail elsewhere (2). The following is a brief summary:

(a) *The medial and lateral PCAs* supply the corresponding half of the choroid. In man the watershed zone between the medial and lateral PCAs may be located anywhere between the fovea and nasal peripapillary choroid (Figure 12.1). The position of the watershed zone is of great clinical significance, since it determines the extent of involvement of the optic nerve head in acute ischemia through occlusion of one of the main PCAs (3).

(b) *The short PCAs:* These supply segments of the choroid extending

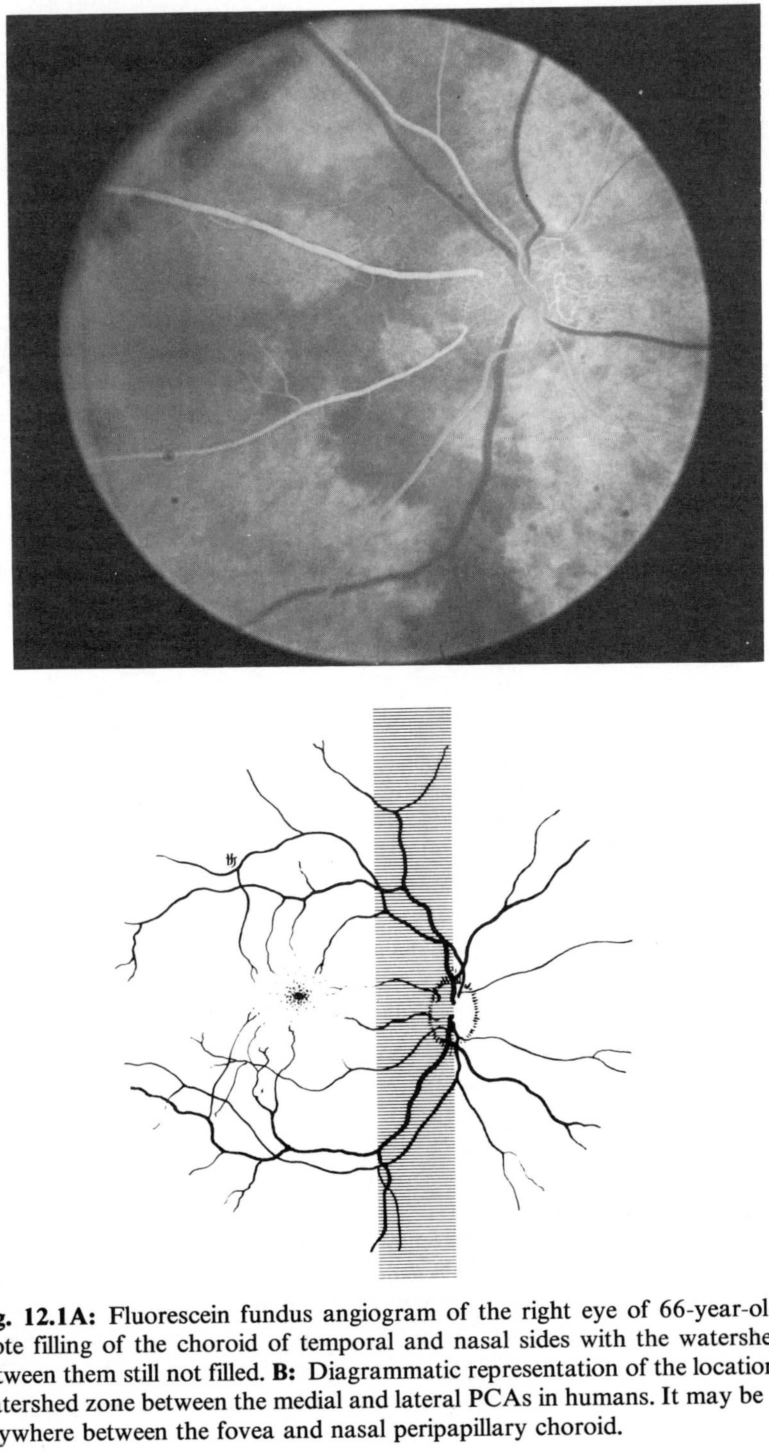

Fig. 12.1A: Fluorescein fundus angiogram of the right eye of 66-year-old man. Note filling of the choroid of temporal and nasal sides with the watershed zone between them still not filled. **B:** Diagrammatic representation of the location of the watershed zone between the medial and lateral PCAs in humans. It may be located anywhere between the fovea and nasal peripapillary choroid.

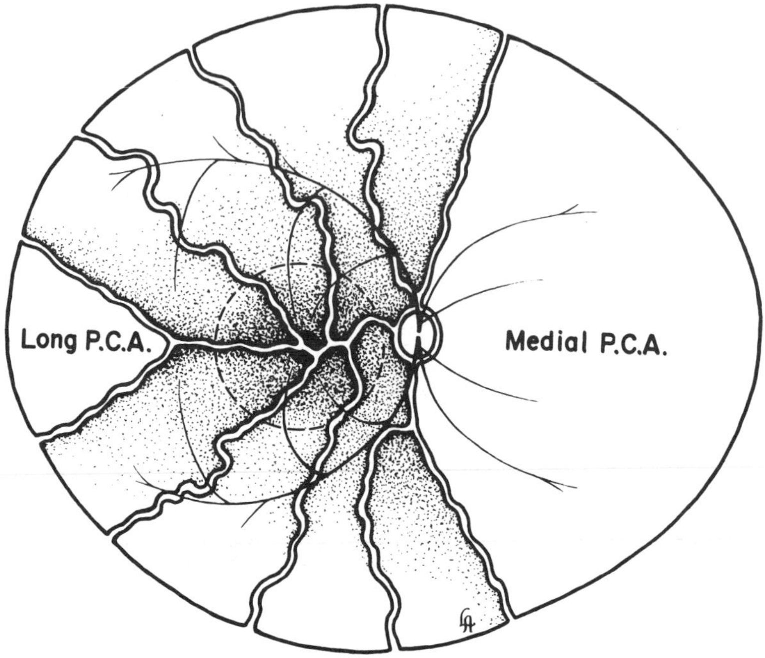

Fig. 12.2. Diagrammatic representation of distribution of various temporal short posterior ciliary arteries (SPCAs) and their watershed zone in posterior part of fundus. Dotted circle in region of distribution of temporal SPCAs represents macular region. Areas of supply by medial PCA and temporal long PCA are also shown.

radially from the posterior pole to the equator; each segment varies greatly in shape, size, and location and has irregular borders (Figure 12.2). Small subdivisions of the short PCAs supply still smaller segments of irregular shape and size, having a geographic pattern. Ultimately, each terminal choroidal arteriole supplies a lobule of choriocapillaris (Figure 12.3).

(c) *The long PCAs:* A detailed account of these arteries is given elsewhere (4). These supply a sector of the choroid extending radially; on the temporal side it extends temporally from the temporal border of the macular region (See figure 12.2).

(d) *Choriocapillaris:* I have given a detailed account of the choriocapillaris elsewhere (5). My fluorescein angiography studies revealed that each terminal choroidal arteriole supplies an independent segment of choriocapillaris, with the arteriole joining the segment in its center and the draining venules lying around the periphery of this segment (Figure 12.3). Each lobule of the choriocapillaris is an independent unit (of a polygonal

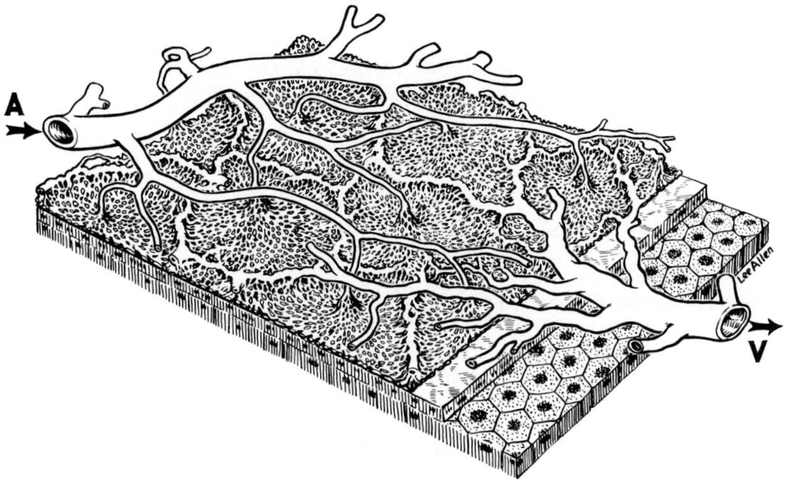

Fig. 12.3. A three-dimensional schematic representation of the choriocapillaris pattern. A, Choroidal arteriole; V, choroidal veins.

shape in the posterior fundus), with no anastomosis with the adjacent segments in vivo. The various segments are arranged like a mosaic, the borders of the mosaic being formed by the venous channels. The size of each lobule of the choriocapillaris varies, and in my studies has been found to be usually about one-quarter of the disc diameter or less.

The in vivo studies thus have indicated that the PCAs and their branches, right down to the terminal choroidal arterioles, and the choriocapillaris have a segmental distribution in the choroid and that the PCAs and choroidal arteries are end-arteries (2).

DISTRIBUTION

The PCAs supply the following:

(a) *Choroid:* as far as the equator.

(b) *Retina:* The choroid supplies the overlying retina to a depth of about 130μ including the retinal pigment epithelium and the adjacent outer layers of the retina up to the outer part of the inner nuclear layer. If a cilioretinal artery is present, then the entire thickness of the retina is supplied in the distribution of the cilio-retinal artery.

(c) *Anterior part of the optic nerve:* The PCA circulation is the main source of blood supply to the optic nerve head and the adjacent retrolaminar part of the optic nerve.

POSTERIOR CILIARY ARTERY OCCLUSION

Our experimental and clinical studies (3, 6–9) have shown that acute occlusion of the PCAs produces the following lesions:

1. Anterior ischemic optic neuropathy
2. Acute choroidal ischemia
3. Cilioretinal artery occlusion, if such an artery exists

Anterior ischemic optic neuropathy

The PCA circulation is the main source of blood supply to the anterior part of the optic nerve. The area of the optic nerve head supplied by the different PCAs shows a marked variation among individuals (3, 10). When there are two PCAs, the entire optic nerve head may be supplied by either the medial or the lateral PCA or the two arteries may share in the supply in varying proportions. When there are three PCAs, they may share the supply of the nerve head. The location of the watershed between the various PCAs in the region of the optic disc (figure 12.1) varies tremendously (see above), and further influences the extent and region of the optic nerve head involved by anterior ischemic optic neuropathy. The importance of the location of the watershed zone lies in the fact that in the event of a fall in the perfusion pressure to the vascular bed supplied by the PCAs, the watershed zone, being an area of comparatively poor vascularity, is most vulnerable to ischemic disorders. Thus, for the production of anterior ischemic optic neuropathy, we do not necessarily require a complete occlusion of the PCAs (3). The subject is discussed elsewhere in detail (3).

Acute choroidal ischemia

The appearance and type of acute choroidal ischemic lesion depend upon the following factors:

(a) *Stage of evolution of the lesions:* Fresh lesions are homogeneously white in color but evolve into chorioretinal pigmentary degenerative lesions within two or three weeks (6).

(b) *Size of the occluded artery or arteriole:* The lesions due to occlusion of large choroidal arteries produce large, triangular, wedge-shaped lesions, with the apex of the wedge toward the posterior pole and the base toward the periphery of the fundus. Those due to occlusion of small arteries or arterioles usually produce geographical lesions of varying sizes, depending upon the size of the occluded vessel. Occlusion of a terminal choroidal arteriole supplying a single lobule of the choriocapillaris produces the so-called Elsching's spot.

(c) *Severity of ischemia:* This may vary from severe, producing complete infarction of the overlying tissue, to mild, producing only a physiological dysfunction, such as breakdown of the chorioretinal barrier of the retinal pigment epithelium, which often results in serous retinal detachment. Very mild choroidal ischemia may produce no visual dysfunction and leave no scars.

Thus, acute choroidal ischemic lesions, because of these variables, have polymorphic presentation but represent a continuous spectrum of disease which is divided into separate entities for descriptive purposes. The available information indicates that Elsching's spot, multifocal acute ischemic choroidopathy (the so-called acute posterior multifocal placoid pigment epitheliopathy), geographic choroidopathy and postoperative acute choroidal ischemia represent some of the conditions (9). If there is a simultaneous obstruction of the choroidal venous circulation, it protects the choroid from acute ischemic effects (8). The subject of acute occlusive disorders of the choroidal vascular bed is discussed at length elsewhere (9).

Cilioretinal Artery Occlusion

If an eye has a cilioretinal artery, in the event of occlusion of its parent PCA, the retina supplied by the cilioretinal artery is infarcted.

ACKNOWLEDGMENT

I am grateful to Mrs. Ellen Ballas for her secretarial help.

REFERENCES

1. Hayreh, S.S.: The ophthalmic artery, III. *Br. J. Ophthalmol.* 46:212, 1962.
2. Hayreh, S.S.: Segmental nature of the choroidal vasculature. *Br. J. Ophthalmol.* 59:631, 1975.
3. Hayreh, S.S.: Anterior ischemic optic neuropathy. Arch. Neurol. 38:675, 1981.
4. Hayreh, S.S.: The long posterior ciliary arteries. Albrecht v. Graefes. *Arch. Ophthalmol.* 192:197, 1974.
5. Hayreh, S.S.: The choriocapillaris. Albrecht v. Graefes. *Arch. Ophthalmol.* 192:165, 1974.
6. Hayreh, S.S., and Baines, J.A.B.: Occlusion of the posterior ciliary artery. II. Chorio-retinal lesions. *Br. J. Ophthalmol.* 56:736, 1972.
7. Hayreh, S.S., and Baines, J.A.B.: Occlusion of the posterior ciliary artery. III. Effects on the optic nerve head. *Br. J. Ophthalmol.* 56:754, 1972.
8. Hayreh, S.S., and Chopdar, A.: Occlusion of the posterior ciliary artery. V. Protective influence of simultaneous vortex vein occlusion. *Arch. Ophthalmol.* 100:1481, 1982.
9. Hayreh, S.S.: Acute occlusive disorders of the choroidal vasculature. *Int. Ophthalmol.* 6:139, 1983.

13

OPTIC NERVE STROKE AND INTERNAL CAROTID ARTERY OCCLUSION

Edward A. Waybright, M.D.

Alterations of perfusion in the carotid artery distribution can cause a number of abnormalities of the visual system. Various retinal changes may occur. In 1960, Hollenhorst (1) discussed ocular signs in a group of 124 patients, 86 with stenosis and 38 with occlusion of the internal carotid artery (ICA). Of these 124 patients, 10 (8%) had unequal hypertensive vascular changes, 15 (12%) unilateral retinopathy (cotten-wool patches), 50 (40%) amaurosis fugax (48 of these 50 patients had stenosis of the ICA), and 21 (17%) retinal infarcts. In 1963, Kearns and Hollenhorst (2) reported venous stasis retinopathy in 5% of patients (22 of 600) with stenosis or occlusion of the ipsilateral ICA. It has subsequently been demonstrated that amaurosis fugax and the majority of retinal infarcts are embolic. Homonymous hemianopia may also be due to emboli. However, prolonged ischemia of the globe can produce other anterior and posterior changes. A grayish cast to the retina, uveitis, iris neovascularization, corneal edema, episcleral vascular injection, and glaucoma were noted by Knox in patients with aortic arch and proximal carotid artery inflammatory involvement (3).

Anterior and posterior optic nerve abnormality most frequently occurs with small blood vessel occlusion. Anterior ischemic optic neuropathy (AION) is characterized by sudden monocular visual loss with ipsilateral disc edema. Visual acuity loss is minimal (20/25) to marked (no light perception), and altitudinal visual field loss in characteristically present. Hypertension occurs in 40 to 50% of patients. Rarely, AION may recur in the same eye. AION is ascribed to occlusion of the short posterior ciliary arteries which perfuse the anterior optic nerve. Anterior ischemic optic neuropathy may be associated with ipsilateral ICA occlusion, but the association is uncommon. The prime differential diagnoses of AION are temporal arteritis and "idiopathic causes." Other causes include vasculitides, sickle cell anemia, migraine, trauma, acute blood loss, internal carotid artery occlusion, and coronary artery bypass graft surgery.

CASE REPORTS

We have reported three patients with AION and ipsilateral ICA occlusion; one also had coronary bypass surgery (4). All three patients had occlusion of the ICA with retrograde flow through the ophthalmic artery filling the middle cerebral artery. The first, a 55-year-old hypertensive woman had sudden onset of blurring of vision in the left eye. On examination she could count fingers on her visual acuity test, and she had disc edema on the left eye. One month later she experienced sudden weakness in her right arm and leg lasting several hours. Optic atrophy was now present on the left and a central scotoma noted on visual field testing. She had mild weakness and sensory loss of the right arm and leg.

The second patient, a 60-year-old hypertensive man with angina had undergone a five vessel coronary artery bypass graft. After surgery he had thoracic bleeding and hypotension. He was reoperated and recovered over the next six days. On the seventh day postoperatively he noticed diminished visual acuity on the right. He had 20/50 visual acuity in the right eye, decreased ability to read color plates, right disc edema, right superior altitudinal visual field defect and a right afferent pupillary defect. He noted numbness in the right hand at the time of visual change.

The third patient was a 48-year-old hypertensive man who presented with blindness of the left eye that had persisted for four days. He had experienced transient right extremity weakness four years earlier. He had no light perception, and left disc edema.

DISCUSSION

Anterior ischemic optic neuropathy with ipsilateral carotid artery disease has been described in single cases by Walsh and Hoyt (5); by Eagling, Saunders and Miller (6); and by Knox and Duke (7), the latter confirmed at autopsy only. AION occurring with coronary bypass was reported by Sweeney et al. (8) in seven patients, two of whom were seen by my colleagues and I. AION associated with acute blood loss was reported by Drance et al. (9) in 1973 and by Hayreh (10) in 1974.

Since decreased perfusion, either selectively in carotid artery distribution or diffusely, may predispose to AION, other possible contributing factors should be considered. Hayreh and Baines have documented a segmental blood supply with a lack of collaterals to the retrolaminar portion of the optic nerve (11). Alm and Bill (12) found limited autoregulation of the distal optic nerve vasculature. In addition to these two inherent limitations of circulation to the distal optic nerve, increased intraocular pressure, atherosclerosis of the short posterior ciliary arteries, or hyalinization of these same vessels due to hypertension could critically reduce perfusion. Retrograde filling of the ophthalmic artery through collaterals of the external carotid artery commonly occurs with ICA occlusion, as found in our patients, and may produce decreased perfusion of the short posterior ciliary arteries. In our patients and others in the literature, multiple factors are often present. Thus, AION could occur with either ICA occlusion alone or ICA occlusion in combination with the other factors noted.

Ischemia of the posterior optic nerve has not been shown to be associated with ICA occlusion. Posterior ischemic optic neuropathy (PION) presents with sudden visual loss, altitudinal or segmental visual field loss and a normal optic disc early. Later, the optic disc atrophies.

Cullen and Duval (13) reported a 71-year-old woman with PION due to atherosclerosis. Hayreh reported a 46-year-old and a 17-year-old with systemic lupus erythematosus and a third patient with temporal arteritis producing a PION. Other references to PION are vague. The posterior optic nerve receives a segmental blood supply from peripheral centripetal vessels by means of a pial plexus. This plexus is said to be supplied by three collateral arteries arising from the ophthalmic artery. The modes of collateral perfusion to the more posterior optic nerve may explain the lack of association of PION with ICA disease, especially ICA occlusion.

CONCLUSIONS

Optic nerve stroke, either anterior or posterior, with ICA stenosis or occlusion is uncommon. However, when symptoms or signs attributable to the appropriate ICA distribution accompany an optic nerve stroke they should be investigated further. Sedimentation rate, other blood studies, noninvasive carotid artery studies and at times, carotid angiography are indicated, if there are signs of ICA disease.

REFERENCES

1. Hollenhorst, R.W.: Significance of bright plaques in the retinal arterioles. *Trans. Am. Ophthalmol. Soc.* 60:316, 1962.
2. Kearns, T.P., Hollenhorst, R.W.: Venous-stasis retinopathy of occlusive disease of the carotid artery. *Proc. Staff Meet. Mayo Clin.* 38:304, 1963.

3. Knox, D.L.: Ischemic ocular inflammation. *Am. J. Ophthalmol.* 60:995, 1965.
4. Waybright, E.A., Selhorst, J.B., and Combs, J.: Anterior ischemic optic neuropathy with internal carotid artery occlusion. *Am. J. Ophthalmol.* 93:42, 1982.
5. Walsh, F.B., Hoyt, W.F.: *Clinical neuro-ophthalmology.* vol 2. Baltimore: Williams and Wilkins, 1979, p. 1828.
6. Eagling, E.M., Saunders, M.D. and Miller, S.J.H.: Ischemic papillopathy. Clinical and fluorescein angiographic review of forty cases. *Br. J. Ophthalmol.* 58:990, 1974.
7. Knox, D.L., Duke, J.R.: Slowly progressive ischemic optic neuropathy. *Trans. Am. Acad. Ophthalmol. Otolaryngol.* 75:1065, 1971.
8. Sweeney, P.J. et al: Ischemic optic neuropathy: a complication of cardiopulmonary bypass surgery. *Neurology* (NY) 32:560, 1982.
9. Drance, S.M., Morgan, R.W., and Sweeney, V.P.: Shock-induced optic neuropathy. *N. Engl. J. Med.* 288:329, 1973.
10. Hayreh, S.S.: Posterior ischemic optic neuropathy. *Ophthalmologica.* 182:29, 1981.
11. Hayreh, S.S., Baines, J.A.B.: Occlusion of the posterior ciliary artery. III. Effects on the optic nerve head. *Br. J. Ophthalmol.* 56:754, 1972.
12. Alm, A., Bill, A.: Ocular and optic nerve blood flow at normal and increased intraocular pressures in monkeys (macaca irus): A study with radioactively labelled microspheres including flow determinations in brain and some other tissues. *Exp. Eye Res.* 15:15, 1973.
13. Cullen, J.F., Duval, J.: Posterior ischemic optic neuropathy (P.I.O.N.). *Neuro-Ophthalmology* 3:15, 1983.

14

EXPERIMENTAL CAROTID ARTERY OCCLUSION

Paul Henkind, M.D., Ph.D.
Gary Korte, Ph.D.
Dan Levy, M.D.
Jason Slakter, M.D.
Alan Spertus, M.D.

During the past two years our group has developed an inexpensive and reproducible model of acute carotid occlusion which produces consistent lesions of the ocular fundus. We have grossly and microscopically examined the short- and long-term fundus alteration induced by carotid artery ligation and have studied the effects of reversing carotid occlusion (1–4). Recently, we have examined the morphologic alterations in the optic nerve induced by our model. In our experiments we have found that unilateral carotid artery occlusion has little or no visible effect upon the fundus although some circulatory changes can be detected by using fluorescein angiography. On the other hand, bilateral carotid occlusion induces significant fundus changes which pursue a predictable course. Restoration of flow through a carotid artery, by removal of the occluder, may improve the fundus picture, but only if the occlusion has been present a relatively short time. This paper reviews our work to date.

MATERIALS AND METHODS

Full details of our methodology have been published (1, 2). We have used, exclusively, healthy Long-Evans pigmented female rats at least one year of age. To the present time we have used 188 rats in order to fulfill our

From the Department of Ophthalmology of the Albert Einstein College of Medicine-Montefiore Medical Center, Bronx, New York.

protocols which required 80 study animals. Anesthesia-related deaths and severe hemorrhage during initial surgery eliminated 72 animals, and the development of cataracts in 36 animals resulted in their exclusion. As our experience increased, the number of anesthesia-related and operative deaths diminished.

The animals were randomly divided into three study groups undergoing either (a) unilateral, (b) bilateral common carotid, or (c) sham ligation. They were further subdivided according to the length of time the ligatures remained in place. When an animal died before completion of the study, its data were discarded and another rat was substituted.

Initially, carotid ligation was accomplished using a 4-0 silk suture tied tightly around the common carotid artery 1 cm proximal to its site of bifurcation. During the later reversal experiments, an 8-mm microvascular clamp was substituted for the silk ligature. All animals had baseline fundus photographs and fluorescein angiograms prior to operation, again at one to two days following carotid surgery, and then at various appropriate intervals during the study.

Ocular tissue for light and electron microscopy as well as retinal digestion was fixed and prepared by routine methods.

Analysis of clinical and histopathological material was done by the group using coded pictures and slides in order to eliminate bias.

OBSERVATIONS AND RESULTS

We will describe the fundus picture as determined from color fundus photographs (Figures 14.1–14.5), then the fluorescein angiographic appearances, and finally the results of histopathological studies. A brief description of our reversibility studies is also provided.

The fundus picture seen at one or two days following either unilateral or sham ligation was generally unremarkable and indistinguishable from baseline evaluations.

Bilaterally ligated animals showed a rather consistent set of abnormalities throughout the experiment. At one or two days post-ligation the following changes were evident: (a) to a varying degree the optic discs appeared blurred and swollen bilaterally; (b) the nerve fiber layer at the posterior pole, normally visible as fine striations radiating from the disc, was totally obscured; (c) the retinal veins were darker appearing than normal, dilated and tortuous, often of irregular caliber, and usually surrounded by a whitish cuff; and (d) the retinal arteries, if initially tortuous became straighter. Sluggish blood flow, demonstrable as “sludging” or “box-carring” was seen in some animals. A single example of superficial retinal hemorrhage in the juxtapapillary region was observed.

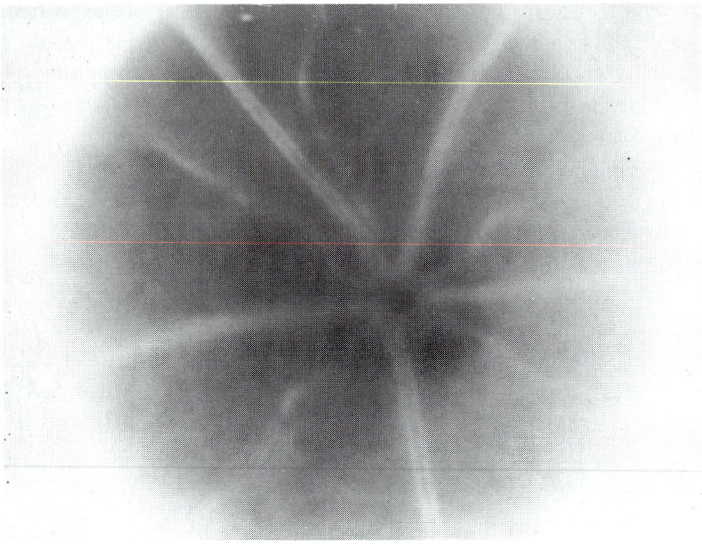

Fig. 14.1. Animal No. 14. Baseline fundus photograph showing normal vasculature along with normal retinal striations.

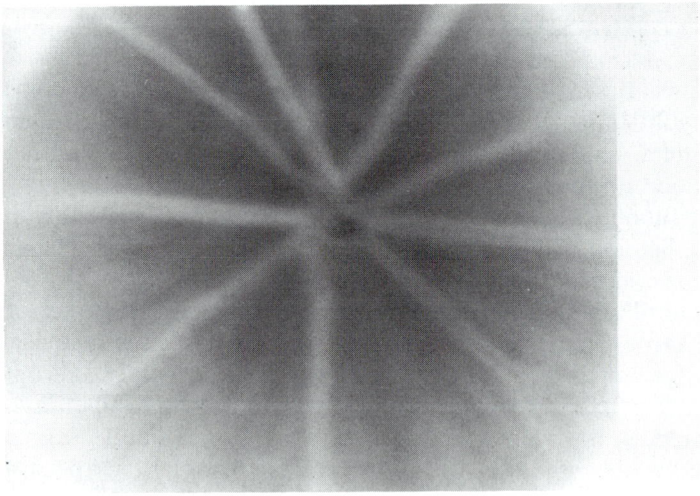

Fig. 14.2. Animal No. 14. Two days following bilateral carotid artery ligation showing swollen optic disc, dilated veins, straightened retinal arterioles, and obscured posterior pole retinal striations.

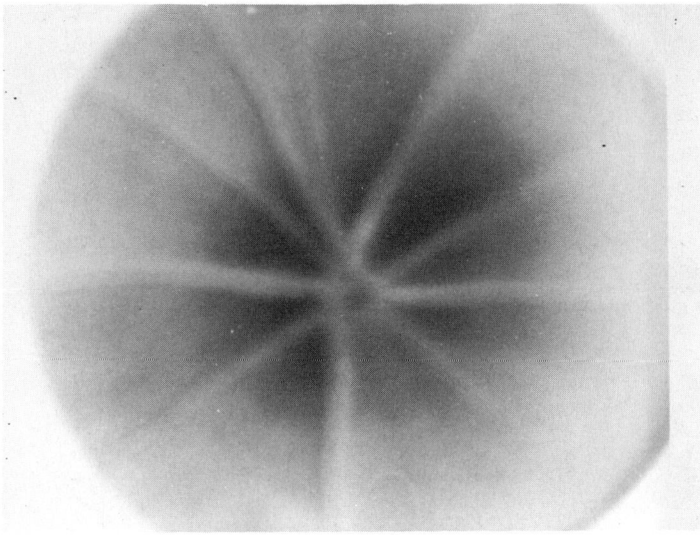

Fig. 14.3. Animal No. 14. One week following bilateral common artery ligation showing decrease in optic disc swelling, less retinal vein dilation, increased arterial light reflex, and diminution of the retinal opacification.

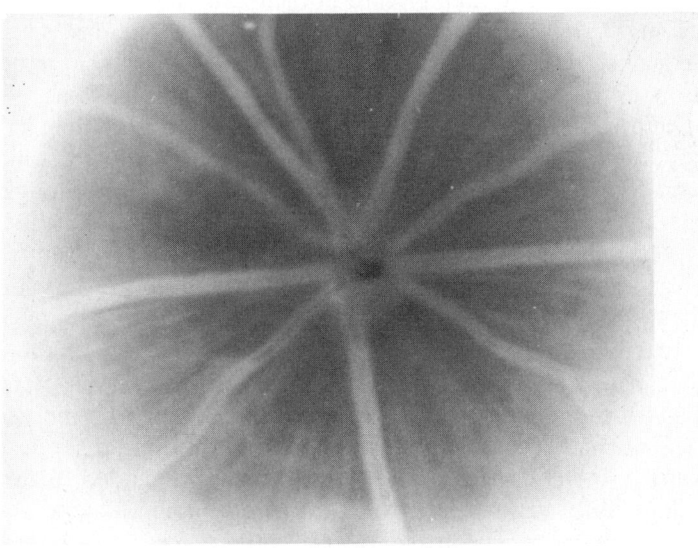

Fig. 14.4. Animal No. 14. Sixteen weeks following bilateral common carotid artery ligation showing peripapillary halo, severe arteriolar constriction, venous narrowing, increased fundus granularity, and absence of the normal nerve fiber layer.

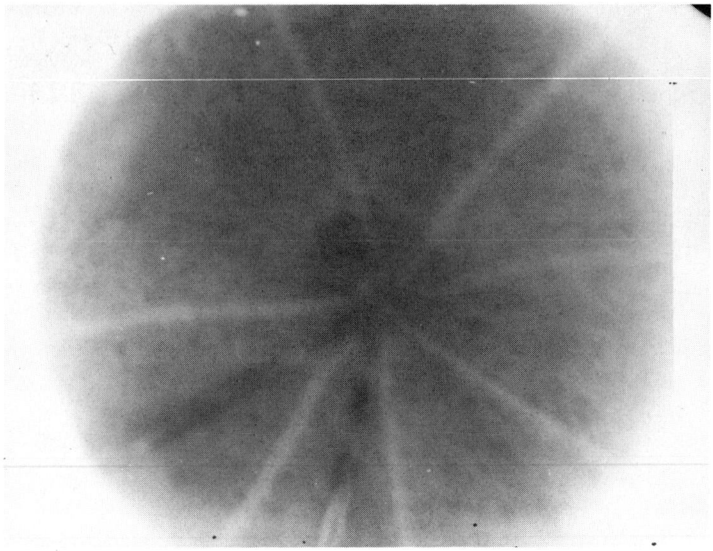

Fig. 14.5. Animal No. 2. Sixteen weeks following bilateral common carotid artery ligation showing marked retinal arteriolar sheathing and a pale disc.

By one week the fundus picture in bilaterally ligated animals showed the following: (a) either persistence or resolution of the disc swelling; (b) continued obscuration of the normal nerve fiber layer pattern, but diminution of the retinal opacification; (c) the retinal veins, while still dilated and tortuous compared to baseline, of lesser caliber then at the two-day study; and (d) the retinal arteries irregular in appearance, some dilated, others constricted, and many with an increased light reflex. Sluggish blood flow was still evident in some vessels. In all animals the white cuffing around vessels, especially veins, had diminished or disappeared. A peripapillary halo was visible in most animals and about one-third had a granular appearance at the posterior pole.

At two weeks the disc swelling had disappeared and there was a prominent peripapillary halo. The vascular changes either persisted or became more pronounced, and most major vessels had an increased light reflex. The normal striated nerve fiber layer pattern had disappeared.

From 2 to 16 weeks consistent changes included a prominent peripapillary halo, venous narrowing towards baseline levels or beyond, varying arterial caliber—some narrowed, others appearing dilated—with an increased light reflex over all but the narrowest arteries, and several examples of marked retinal arterial sheathing (Figure 14.5). Increased fundus granularity and an absence of the normal nerve fiber layer were constant features.

protocols which required 80 study animals. Anesthesia-related deaths and severe hemorrhage during initial surgery eliminated 72 animals, and the development of cataracts in 36 animals resulted in their exclusion. As our experience increased, the number of anesthesia-related and operative deaths diminished.

The animals were randomly divided into three study groups undergoing either (a) unilateral, (b) bilateral common carotid, or (c) sham ligation. They were further subdivided according to the length of time the ligatures remained in place. When an animal died before completion of the study, its data were discarded and another rat was substituted.

Initially, carotid ligation was accomplished using a 4-0 silk suture tied tightly around the common carotid artery 1 cm proximal to its site of bifurcation. During the later reversal experiments, an 8-mm microvascular clamp was substituted for the silk ligature. All animals had baseline fundus photographs and fluorescein angiograms prior to operation, again at one to two days following carotid surgery, and then at various appropriate intervals during the study.

Ocular tissue for light and electron microscopy as well as retinal digestion was fixed and prepared by routine methods.

Analysis of clinical and histopathological material was done by the group using coded pictures and slides in order to eliminate bias.

OBSERVATIONS AND RESULTS

We will describe the fundus picture as determined from color fundus photographs (Figures 14.1–14.5), then the fluorescein angiographic appearances, and finally the results of histopathological studies. A brief description of our reversibility studies is also provided.

The fundus picture seen at one or two days following either unilateral or sham ligation was generally unremarkable and indistinguishable from baseline evaluations.

Bilaterally ligated animals showed a rather consistent set of abnormalities throughout the experiment. At one or two days post-ligation the following changes were evident: (a) to a varying degree the optic discs appeared blurred and swollen bilaterally; (b) the nerve fiber layer at the posterior pole, normally visible as fine striations radiating from the disc, was totally obscured; (c) the retinal veins were darker appearing than normal, dilated and tortuous, often of irregular caliber, and usually surrounded by a whitish cuff; and (d) the retinal arteries, if initially tortuous became straighter. Sluggish blood flow, demonstrable as "sludging" or "box-carring" was seen in some animals. A single example of superficial retinal hemorrhage in the juxtapapillary region was observed.

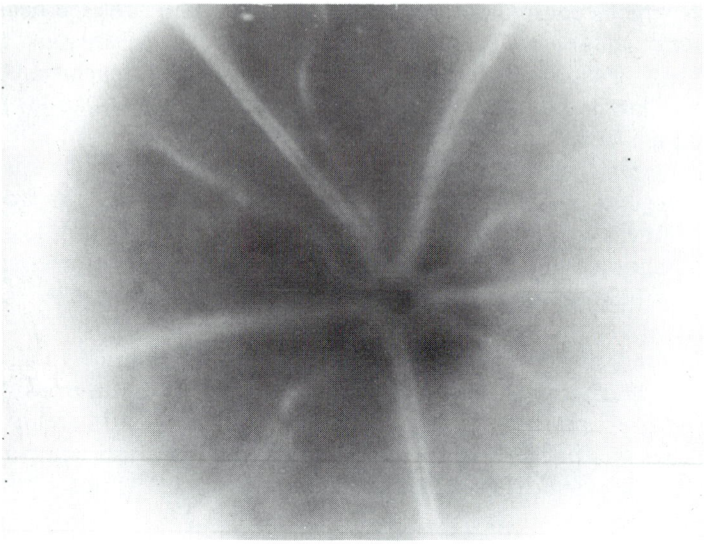

Fig. 14.1. Animal No. 14. Baseline fundus photograph showing normal vasculature along with normal retinal striations.

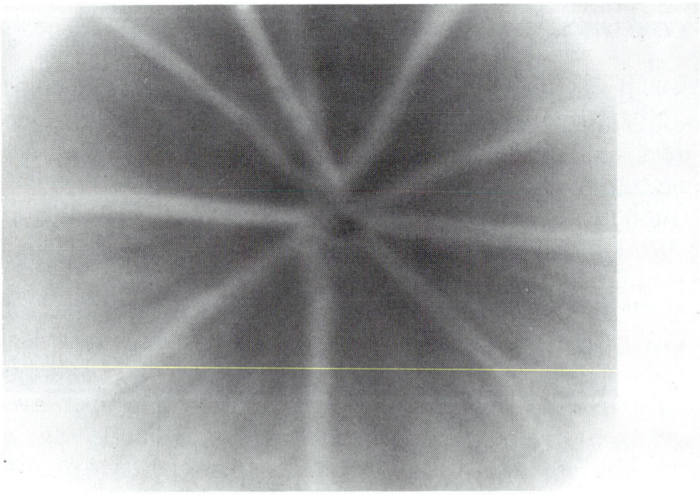

Fig. 14.2. Animal No. 14. Two days following bilateral carotid artery ligation showing swollen optic disc, dilated veins, straightened retinal arterioles, and obscured posterior pole retinal striations.

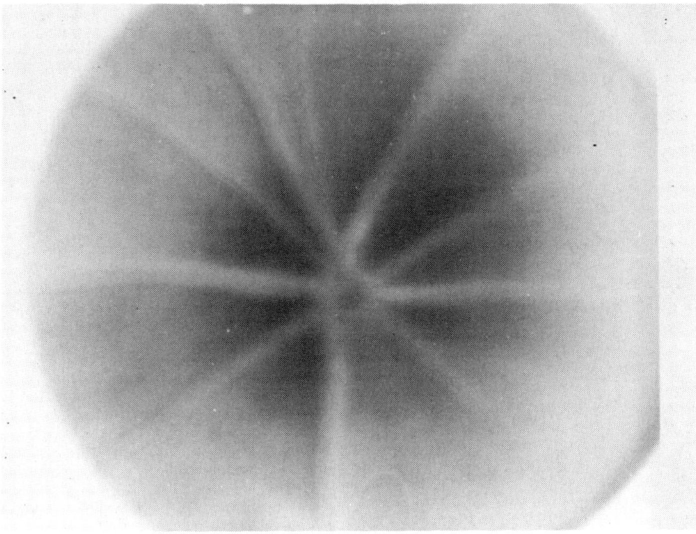

Fig. 14.3. Animal No. 14. One week following bilateral common artery ligation showing decrease in optic disc swelling, less retinal vein dilation, increased arterial light reflex, and diminution of the retinal opacification.

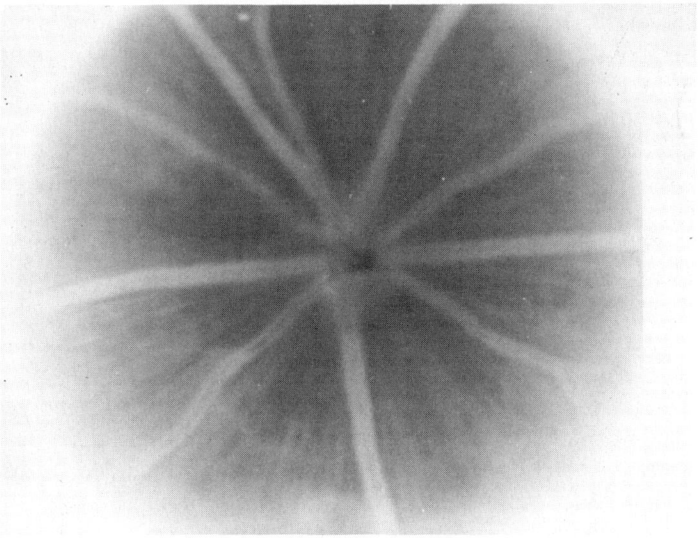

Fig. 14.4. Animal No. 14. Sixteen weeks following bilateral common carotid artery ligation showing peripapillary halo, severe arteriolar constriction, venous narrowing, increased fundus granularity, and absence of the normal nerve fiber layer.

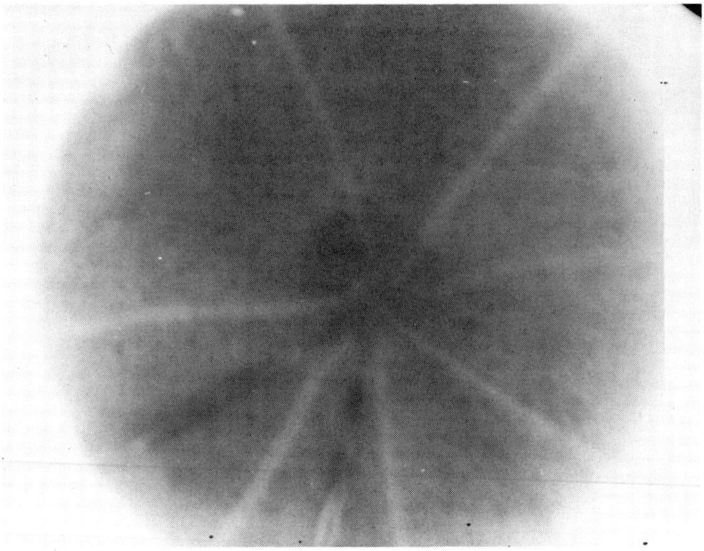

Fig. 14.5. Animal No. 2. Sixteen weeks following bilateral common carotid artery ligation showing marked retinal arteriolar sheathing and a pale disc.

By one week the fundus picture in bilaterally ligated animals showed the following: (a) either persistence or resolution of the disc swelling; (b) continued obscuration of the normal nerve fiber layer pattern, but diminution of the retinal opacification; (c) the retinal veins, while still dilated and tortuous compared to baseline, of lesser caliber then at the two-day study; and (d) the retinal arteries irregular in appearance, some dilated, others constricted, and many with an increased light reflex. Sluggish blood flow was still evident in some vessels. In all animals the white cuffing around vessels, especially veins, had diminished or disappeared. A peripapillary halo was visible in most animals and about one-third had a granular appearance at the posterior pole.

At two weeks the disc swelling had disappeared and there was a prominent peripapillary halo. The vascular changes either persisted or became more pronounced, and most major vessels had an increased light reflex. The normal striated nerve fiber layer pattern had disappeared.

From 2 to 16 weeks consistent changes included a prominent peripapillary halo, venous narrowing towards baseline levels or beyond, varying arterial caliber—some narrowed, others appearing dilated—with an increased light reflex over all but the narrowest arteries, and several examples of marked retinal arterial sheathing (Figure 14.5). Increased fundus granularity and an absence of the normal nerve fiber layer were constant features.

Though we searched for them, we found no examples of disc or retinal neovascularization or collateral vessel formation.

Fluorescein angiography proved to be a more sensitive indicator of the vascular changes, since it provided information about circulation time as well as permeability alterations. In animals treated by sham operation there were no angiographic findings that deviated from normal baseline. A few of the unilaterally ligated animals showed a slight delay in circulation time through the retina and some venous dilation at 24 or 48 hours. Such changes occurred in only one-third of the animals. From 1 to 16 weeks the delay in circulation time, if previously noted, might persist as did some irregularities in vessel caliber.

All bilaterally ligated animals exhibited marked changes in their fluorescein angiograms. At 24 or 48 hours following operation it was noted that disc fluorescence preceded retinal arterial infilling, a situation opposite to that noted in most baseline studies. There was disc edema evidenced by disc hyperfluorescence and marked slowing of retinal circulation time. Retinal arterial infilling was delayed as was filling of the retinal veins, and there was gross irregularity of the normal capillary bed pattern.

By one week, the early disc fluorescence and the late peripapillary staining and leakage had diminished or resolved. Retinal circulation time was still slower than normal, venous dilation, quite prominent initially, was slightly reduced, but the capillary bed maintained a coarse pattern. In about one-half of the animals, major vessels had an irregular caliber. There was a patchy appearance to the choroidal pattern, and a distinct peripapillary halo was seen.

By two weeks the disc edema and venous dilation had completely resolved in all animals, but the remainder of the abnormalities noted at one week persisted. From 2 to 16 weeks the fluorescein angiographic appearances remained essentially unchanged.

Light and electron microscopic studies have been conducted on specimens ranging from 2 days to 16 weeks post-ligation. Few or no abnormalities have been seen in the retinas or optic nerves of unilateral or sham ligated animals.

By two days after operation the bilaterally ligated animals had severe degenerative changes visible both by light and electron microscopy. Such changes were most evident in the inner retina. There were changes in the nerve fiber, inner nuclear, and inner plexiform layers. By one week after ligation, the neurons in these layers appeared normal except for scattered cells and processes undergoing the type of degeneration termed *dark degeneration* by neurocytologists. By two weeks post-ligation these inner layers appeared similar to controls, though some dark degenerating cells and processes still could be found. These were thought to belong primarily to horizontal or bipolar cells.

At 16 weeks post-ligation the inner retinal layers were very thin. However, there were large expanses of normal-appearing nervous tissue.

With regard to photoreceptors, only mild degeneration was visible two days to two weeks post-ligation. However, at 16 weeks the photoreceptor terminals showed severe degeneration. It appeared that the photoreceptor degeneration was a slower process than the degeneration noted for the inner retinal cells.

To date, by routine light or electron microscopy we have not observed any significant changes in retinal or choroidal vessels, especially capillaries. However, as noted below, such changes were found on retinal digestion studies.

Mild changes in the retinal pigment epithelium were seen in some long-term specimens, but these require further analysis.

With regard to optic nerve changes, we have studied rats treated with bilateral ligation as well as controls (5). Controls had no pathological findings. All of the others, followed for 16 weeks, were noted to have a normal circle of Willis on brain examination using an operating microscope. In every instance they had marked atrophy of their optic nerves which were reduced in size from one-third to one-half normal diameter. Ultrastructural analysis revealed loss of both myelinated and unmyelinated optic nerve axons, replacement of normal tissue by astrocytes, and macrophages which contained myelin and other degradation products.

Examination of retinal digest preparations showed no differences between sham or unilaterally ligated animals and normals (3). The situation with regard to bilaterally ligated animals was quite different and significant changes were always found. First, it appeared that the number of intramural pericytes was increased in this group compared to normals, and this occurred in all three retinal zones, peripapillary, mid-retinal, and peripheral. The ratio of endothelial cell to intramural pericyte nuclei was markedly decreased in the retinal periphery. Secondly, with regard to acellular strands there was a marked increase in the number of thick acellular strands compared to normals (Figure 14.6). While the greatest number of such strands was found in the peripapillary region, the most significant difference between the number of these strands in the bilaterally ligated animals, compared to sham and unilaterally ligated animals, was noted in the retinal periphery.

With regard to reversibility of fundus changes after removal of the carotid occlusion, we have studied 24 animals who had bilateral microvascular clamps placed at initial surgery. Twelve of these animals had one clamp removed either at one, two, or four weeks and another twelve had both clamps removed at one, two, or four weeks. Removal of one clamp at one week resulted in ipsilateral reversibility of the vascular changes in three of four rats, while removal of both clamps at one week resulted in bilateral reversibility in three of four animals. No visible improvement could be seen when clamps were removed at two weeks. In all of these animals we felt that there was restoration of carotid blood flow. In animals whose clamps were removed at four weeks or beyond, there was no ocular change noted and no restoration in carotid blood flow.

DISCUSSION

We developed the present model of carotid occlusion in order to ascertain whether we could mimic or duplicate the fundus findings alleged to occur in human carotid artery occlusive disease. Oddly, it is only relatively recently that there has been an appreciation of what carotid artery occlusion may produce in the fundus, exclusive of embolic effects from diseased but not occluded carotid arteries (4–6). The term *venous-stasis retinopathy*, coined by Kearns and Hollenhorst in 1963 (4), would seem appropriate for the clinical picture they viewed and would not be inappropriate for the condition we have produced in rats with bilaterally occluded carotid arteries. Certainly, the most dramatic vascular change induced appeared to be on the venous side of the retinal circulation. Here we found dark veins which undoubtedly reflect reduced blood flow and diminished oxygen content within the lumen of the veins. Their dilation and tortuosity suggest some inherent autoregulatory property and elasticity. One major difference between the human and rat fundus is the lack of arteriovenous crossings at the posterior pole in the rat. In the human situation tortuosity may be more apparent because of the tethering that occurs at such crossings.

Irregularities in the retinal arteries reflect changes in blood flow and presumably are dictated by autoregulation. The term autoregulation is loosley used and basically reflects the fact that retinal vessels lack intrinsic nerves, suggesting that the vessels contract or dilate due to an internal mechanism residing within the vessel itself. The increased light reflex which was noted over arteries and veins in our chronic animals suggests that the walls of the vessels have undergone alterations similar to those seen in human arteriosclerosis. Sheathing of the retinal arteries seen in some chronic animals must certainly indicate profound vascular wall pathology. Normally, retinal vessels are transparent and only the blood column is visible. We have yet to study the ultrastructural characteristics of the rat retinal arteries and veins in normal, compared to chronically ligated animals. We intend to do this in conjunction with studies of retinal vessels in hypertensive rats.

We found only a single example of a retinal hemorrhage in one animal, no microaneurysms or retinal neovascularization, and no persistent

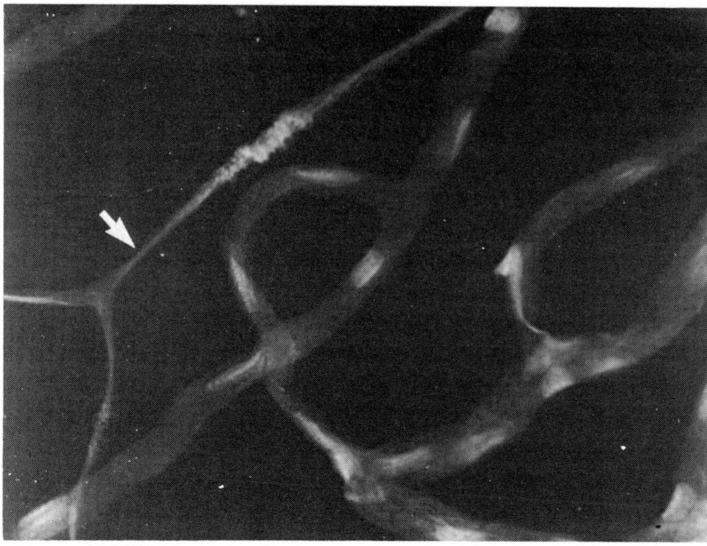

Fig. 14.6. Retinal digest showing thick acellular strands (*arrow*).

exudates. Perhaps such alterations might have occured if the animals had been maintained for a longer duration, but we doubt this. Indeed, we were struck by the fact that the major vascular alterations tended to spontaneously resolve, at least to some extent, in chronically ligated animals. Conceivably this may occur in humans as well.

The fact that fundus findings in humans may be reversed by surgery to reestablish carotid artery flow (7, 8) has been confirmed by our experiments with reversal. However, we were only successful when the occlusion was relieved within a week of ligation.

Quite significant, we believe, are the results of examining retinal digest preparations. The fact that experimental carotid occlusion caused no alterations in unilaterally ligated animals and consistent capillary bed alterations in bilaterally treated animals raises a number of questions. First, is unilateral carotid occlusion generally of little consequence for the retina? Since both humans and rats possess a circle of Willis, good arterial perfusion may readily occur even if one carotid is totally obstructed. The finding of fundus alterations suggestive of carotid occlusion points strongly to bilateral occlusion or, possibly, poor collateral circulation. Secondly, once the retinal circulation is markedly compromised, the major alterations may be at a vascular level invisible to ophthalmoscopy, but visible on fluorescein angiography and retinal digestion. Do some retinal capillaries "drop out" in order for others to survive? That is a vital question with implications for the entire central nervous system if it is faced with decreased arterial perfusion.

One facet of our work that requires more study concerns the edematous appearance of the optic nerve head and the posterior pole retina which occurred shortly after bilateral carotid artery occlusion. We feel that this may represent embarrassed axoplasmic flow in the inner retinal layers, especially the nerve fiber layer, and thus may be analogous to the cotton-wool spots that may occur in venous-stasis retinopathy. The spontaneous resolution of this feature even when the ligation is maintained is not surprising since cotton-wool spots in humans resolve by themselves. The fact that in an early stage the fundus picture in rats revealed cuffing most prominent around major posterior pole veins would be in line with the idea that the most hypoxic retinal area would be abutting the veins and here axoplasmic flow derangement, if secondary to hypoxia, would be most profound.

The peripapillary atrophy consistently noted in chronically ligated animals simply reflects the marked atrophy of the optic nerve which we have demonstrated histologically. The mottled appearance to the posterior pole may reflect subtle damage to the retinal pigment epithelium, and this has been hinted at in our histologic preparations.

CONCLUSIONS

The model we report is useful and inexpensive, and in some ways resembles a spontaneous human disorder. It is not suggested that it totally mimics the condition in humans. One aspect that may make it more useful is to occlude each common carotid artery over a time interval of several weeks rather than at the same time as the operation. Humans likely develop their condition over a lengthy period of time with first one and then the other artery becoming blocked. We are aware of the fact that in humans marked, but not total, obstruction of the carotid leaves little evidence in the eye, and it may not be until total sudden occlusion occurs that any ocular manifestation is expressed. Thus, the sudden occlusion experimentally induced may not be far off target for what actually takes place in humans.

A feature of this work that may not be readily recognizable is the fact that much of the study was conducted by third and fourth year medical students during their elective and spare time. They not only learned a wide variety of sophisticated clinical and laboratory techniques but they also found out that research can be rewarding for its own sake.

ACKNOWLEDGMENTS

We would like to thank Noel Roa, Mary Ellen Murphy, Ken Kostuk, and Larry Egan for their expert assistance during the conduct of this work. Supported in part by an unrestricted grant from Research to Prevent Blindness, Inc., The Coyne Scholarship Award, the Edward Goodman Memorial Fund (all for Dr. Levy), a Neil Weisman Award from Fight for Sight, Inc., and the Education and Research Fund of the Department of Ophthalmology of the Albert Eintein College of Medicine.

REFERENCES

1. Slakter, J.S., Spertus, A.D., Weissman, S.S. and Henkind, P.: An experimental model of carotid artery occlusive disease. *Am. J. Ophthalmol.* 97:168, 1984.
2. Spertus, A.D., Slakter, J.S., Weissman, S.S. and Henkind, P.: Experimental carotid occlusion: funduscopic and fluorescein angiographic findings. *Brit. J. Ophthalmol.* 68:47, 1984.
3. Glatt, H.J., Henkind, P.: Aging changes in the retinal capillary bed of the rat. *Microvasc. Res.* 18:1, 1979.
4. Kearns, T.P., Hollenhorst, R.W.: Venous-stasis retinopathy of occlusive disease of the carotid artery. *Proc. Staff Meet. Mayo Clin.* 38:304, 1963.
5. Hedges, T.R., Jr.: Ophthalmoscopic findings in internal carotid occlusion. *Am. J. Ophthalmol.* 55:1007, 1963.
6. Kearns, T.P.: Ophthalmology and the carotid artery. *Am. J. Ophthalmol.* 88:714, 1979.
7. Neupert, J.R., Brubaker, R.F., Kearns, T.P., and Sundt, T.M.: Rapid resolution of venous stasis retinopathy after carotid endarterectomy. *Am. J. Ophthalmol.* 81:600, 1976.
8. Kearns, T.P., Younge, B.R., and Piepgras, D.G.: Resolution of venous stasis retinopathy after carotid artery bypass surgery. *Mayo Clin. Proc.* 55:342, 1980.

15

SEVERE ISCHEMIC SYNDROMES OF THE RETINA AND OPTIC NERVE AND THEIR PROBABLE CAROTID ORIGINS

Ramon Berguer, M.D., Ph.D.

Most visual loss problems referred to vascular surgeons for workup of carotid disease are either transient, as in amaurosis fugax, or partial, as in retinal branch artery occlusion. Patients with more severe total infarcts of the retina, such as in central retinal artery occlusion, or of the head of the optic nerve are seldom suspected of carotid disease and, in the latter case, are generally labeled *idiopathic*. Ophthalmologists routinely refer patients with partial and transient visual loss to vascular surgeons, but generally view massive infarcts of the retina or optic nerve as an end-stage problem.

If comparisons are made to other organs and territories, one may draw the conclusion that acute massive ischemia is generally the consequence of the occlusion of an important vessel by an embolus or thrombus. The oft-quoted and ill-defined "small vessel disease" often blamed for these catastrophic infarcts in the retina or optic nerve represents a minority of the acute problems encountered in the practice of vascular surgery in any territory.

It is intriguing that vascular surgeons see so many patients with embolic disease of the branches of the central retinal artery (CRA), relatively few with central retinal artery occlusion (CRAO) and very few with ischemia of the optic nerve head. This is all the more curious because the CRA and its branches, as well as the posterior ciliary arteries (PCAs) supplying the optic nerve head, all derive their supply from the same source, the ophthalmic artery.

Why would segmental retinal ischemia so often be due to embolization while CRAO and ischemia of the optic nerve head so often be called idiopathic? Perhaps the explanation is that we can *see* the emboli in the retinal branches, but have no way to observe what has happened to the CRA or PCAs in their intraorbital course.

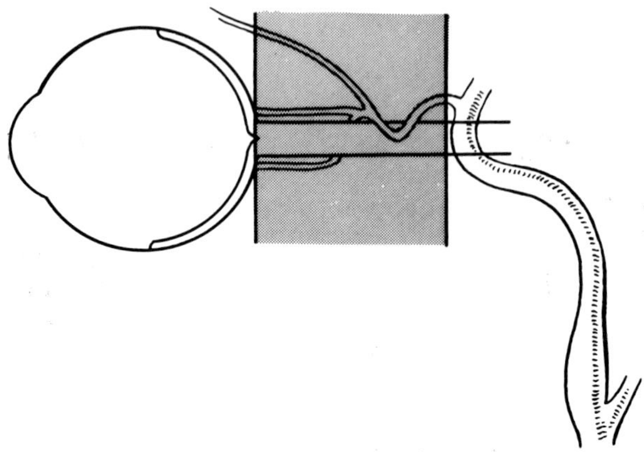

Fig. 15.1. Arterial supply to the eye: the gray area of illiteracy.

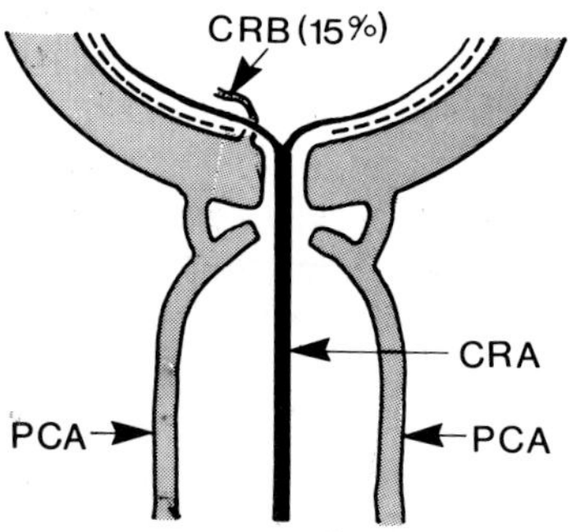

Fig. 15.2. Schematic drawings of the CRA and PCA supply.

ANATOMY OF THE ORBITAL VASCULATURE

Little information exists in the literature about the anatomy of the orbital vasculature and even less about its pathology. The ophthalmologist's interest fades behind the retina and that of the vascular surgeon ends at the carotid siphon. The blood supply of the optic nerve and eyeball travels through the orbit, but this supply is barely visible in standard angiograms. Furthermore, postmortem studies have traditionally avoided the orbit and, as a result, the contents of this inaccessible cavity fall into a gray area of near illiteracy (Figure 15.1).

Both the central retinal artery and posterior ciliary arteries are branches of the ophthalmic artery (Figure 15.2). The CRA travels inside the optic nerve and supplies the retina. It has a diameter of approximately 0.3 mm. The PCAs are a bit larger, about 0.5 mm in diameter, and, in addition to the choroid, they supply the head of the optic nerve. In 15% of the population the PCAs send a small cilioretinal branch which supplies a small segment of retina. In this small minority, the cilioretinal branches can be seen by ophthalmoscopy and by intravenous fluorescein angiography.

Nor is the CRA visible with the resolution obtained in today's x-ray equipment. The PCAs on the contrary can be seen in magnified views although they are often difficult to identify positively because of overlap of branches of the external carotid arteries, and sometimes, too, because of their faint filling when there is a severe carotid stenosis proximally.

The incidence of embolization to a distal vessel is determined by its caliber in relation to the size of the embolizing particle and by its flow rate. Small particle embolization of the CRA and its branches is fairly common, but because of their larger size, embolization of the PCAs should be more frequent than that of the CRA. The symptoms of PCA occlusion, however, may not always have the striking clinical findings of a retinal branch occlusion because they are not "terminal" arteries as is the CRA.

The work of Hayreh (see chapters 6 and 12) has shown the similarity between the ophthalmological findings in ischemic optic neuropathy and those observed in monkeys whose PCAs had been occluded. Unfortunately, in ischemic optic neuropathy, the ophthalmoscope reveals the consequences rather than the cause of optic nerve ischemia. The tenuous arterial supply of the optic nerve head can only be evaluated by special arteriographic techniques. We know little about the pathological changes in these PCAs.

We have little information about this area, also, because postmortem examinations of the orbit have been discouraged by social custom and thus avoided by investigators. But looking closely at the analogies in other parts of the body, it appears that the use of the term *idiopathic* in reference to most optic nerve strokes begs the question of their etiology. There is, indeed, no reason to reject the sensible hypothesis that ischemic infarction of the optic nerve head has the same embolic or thrombotic cause that we observe in other parts of the brain.

CLINICAL FINDINGS

A high incidence of carotid artery disease in patients presenting with sudden changes in vision has been noted. To highlight this correlation, let me refer to a pilot study we conducted that included 20 patients with acute ophthalmological findings in 20 symptomatic eyes. The average age was 63 years with the range from 47 to 91 years of age. The male-to-female ratio was 0.8. These patients were seen over a period of two years by both the Department of Ophthalmology and the Section of Vascular Surgery. The aims of the project were:

TABLE 15.1. Distribution of arterial pathology in the 20 patients examined

Central retinal art. system	
CRA occlusion	7
Cholesterol embolus	4
Amaurosis fugax	3
Posterior ciliary art. system	
Ischemic optic neuropathy	3
Cilio-retinal branch occ.	2
Others	
Venous stasis	1
Total patients/eyes	20

1. To study the vascular anatomy of the orbit in patients with acute ischemic events of the retina or optic nerve.
2. To investigate the incidence of carotid pathology in these patients.
3. To study the incidence of arterial disease in the opposite carotid and orbital vessels.

These patients underwent four-vessel arteriography, including visualization of the arch of the aorta, selective injections of both carotid and subclavian arteries, and magnified orbital views. When indicated, they had intravenous fluorescein angiography in addition to a standard ophthalmological examination.

Fourteen eyes showed evidence of ischemia in the CRA system: seven had CRA occlusion, four had a cholesterol embolus in one of the branches of the CRA. Three patients with amaurosis fugax had normal eye findings. Five patients had findings consistent with ischemia of the PCA system: three had ischemic optic neuropathy and two had occlusion of a cilioretinal branch. One other patient presenting with venous stasis retinopathy could not be assigned to either group (Table 15.1).

Arteriographic Findings

We then reviewed the ipsilateral arteriographic findings in those ischemic eyes (Table 15.2). Twelve patients had internal carotid artery lesions, for an incidence of 60%. In two of these patients, the internal carotid was occluded. In five of the 20 sides (25%), we found ophthalmic artery disease. In five patients magnified views did not visualize the PCA on the symptomatic side. In two of the patients other unrelated vascular lesions were found, namely an aneurysm of the middle cerebral artery and

TABLE 15.2. Ipsilateral and contralateral arteriographic findings in this series

Condition	*Ratio*	*%*
Ipsilateral		
Internal carotid disease	12/20 (2 occluded)	60
Ophthalmic artery lesions	5/20	25
Non-visualization PCA	5/20	25
Other lesions	2/20	10
Contralateral		
Internal carotid disease	10/20	50
Ophthalmic artery lesions	1/20	5

Arteriographic findings in 20 ischemic symptomatic eyes.

an external carotid-to-vertebral artery steal from proximal subclavian artery stenosis.

Patients with severe or symptomatic carotid disease of one side have a high incidence of contralateral carotid lesions. We looked at the carotid arteries in the asymptomatic side and found that 10 out of 20 patients had disease in the opposite carotid system. One patient had ophthalmic artery disease in the contralateral asymptomatic side.

Concomitant medical conditions (Table 15.3) in the 20 patients studied included a high incidence of hypertension, coronary artery disease, and diabetes, which is consistent with what is usually found in a general population of vascular patients. Only one patient had hyperactive platelets in the absence of arterial disease. Platelet aggregation and electron microscopy morphology studies were done after we failed to show an arterial cause for ischemic disease of the eye. Such studies were not conducted in patients who already demonstrated a likely source for their problem, so this single case may represent an underestimate of the true incidence of platelet abnormalities in this group of patients.

In patients presenting with amaurosis fugax, the incidence of operable carotid artery disease is very high, around 90%. In this group of patients with ischemic disease of the eye, the incidence of carotid operations was lower, but still a substantial 40%.

DISCUSSION

The incidence of carotid disease among patients with ischemic disease of the eye is 60% for the symptomatic side and 50% for the opposite side. A similarly high incidence of bilaterality in carotid lesions is found in the general atherosclerotic population. Ischemic optic neuropathy is also often

TABLE 15.3. Concomitant medical conditions (20 patients)

Condition	*Ratio*	*%*
Hypertension	11/20	55
Coronary artery disease	8/20	40
Diabetes	5/20	25
Increased ESR	3/20	15
Lipid/cholesterol abn.	3/20	15
Sticky platelets	1/20	5

bilateral, though not often simultaneously so. The question arises, is this because of intrinsic and bilateral disease of the PCA or because the likely source of emboli, the carotid bifurcation, is often bilaterally diseased?

Finding lesions in the ophthalmic artery on the symptomatic side in 25% of patients was a surprise. One patient had narrowing of the distal half of the vessel (Figure 15.3), three had a stenosis at the takeoff of the ophthalmic artery (Figure 15.4), and two had infundibular aneurysms of the origin of the vessel (Figure 15.5). We do not know if the ophthalmic artery stenosis played any role in the eye symptoms because the patients with this finding also had carotid bifurcation disease. It is worth noting that the two patients with infundibular aneurysms had no other evidence of atherosclerotic disease of their arteriogram. Since arterial aneurysms are a common source of emboli in other locations, perhaps the aneurysm was the embolic source in these two cases.

Available evidence suggests that ischemic disease of the retina and of the optic nerve head is probably due in most cases to embolization from lesions in the carotid, or, less frequently, the ophthalmic arteries.

We are now engaged in a prospective study of patients with ischemic eye problems, which will include arteriography, fluorescein angiography, and detailed orbital arteriography to improve resolution of the PCA outline. In addition we will test these patients for evidence of any of the other suggested etiologies. Long-term follow-up studies of the opposite eye and the carotid artery will also help to clarify whether the bilaterality of ischemic optic neuropathy is secondary to intrinsic disease of the PCA or rather to embolic disease from the opposite carotid artery.

In light of our experience, we suggest that patients with ischemic problems of the retina or optic nerve head should be studied by four-vessel arteriography to delineate both carotid and ophthalmic arteries, since evidence points to these arteries as the source of embolization of the CRA and PCA. The angiographic detail needed can only be provided with selective intraarterial studies and should include magnified orbital views. If a plaque or ulceration is found in the ipsilateral carotid, an endarterectomy

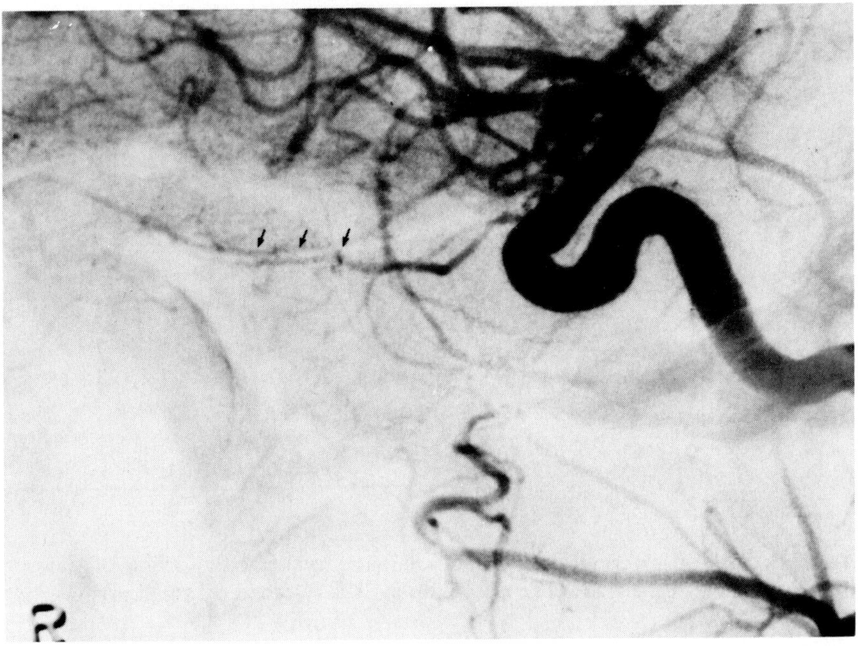

Fig. 15.3. Orbital arteriogram showing narrowing of the distal half of the ophthalmic artery (*arrows*).

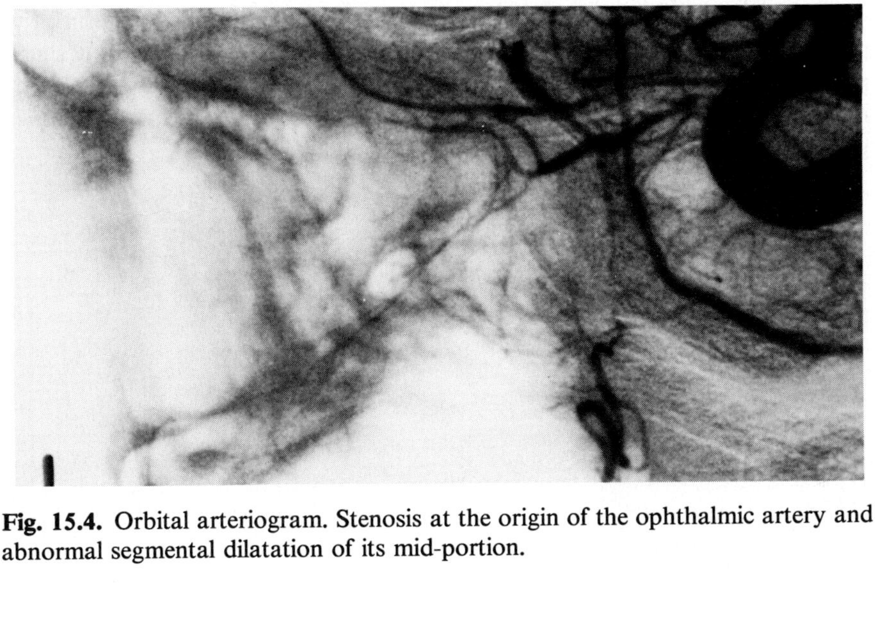

Fig. 15.4. Orbital arteriogram. Stenosis at the origin of the ophthalmic artery and abnormal segmental dilatation of its mid-portion.

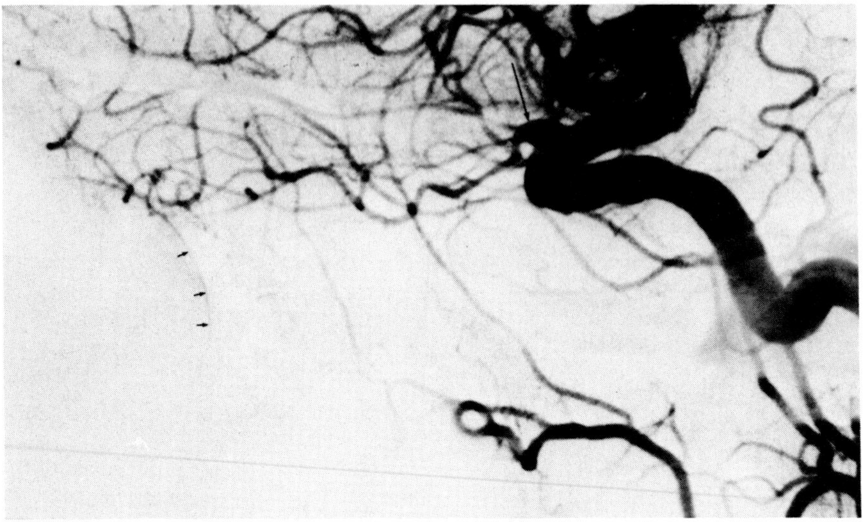

Fig. 15.5. Orbital arteriogram. Infundibular aneurysm at the origin of the ophthalmic artery (*long arrow*). The choroid plexus is outlined by small arrows.

is advisable, provided that the combined mortality and morbidity record of the operating surgeon is under 2% for this operation.

Closer cooperation between ophthalmologic and vascular surgeons is needed to define precisely the relationship between ischemic eye syndromes and disease of the carotid arterial system. It would be useful to redefine the various ischemic syndromes of the eye, abandoning purely descriptive terms and integrating these syndromes with the known mechanics and pathogenesis of arterial deterioration. Going from description to mechanism is the first step for the institution of rational treatment of these problems.

16

CENTRAL RETINAL ARTERY OCCLUSION: TREATMENT BY RETROGRADE SUPRAORBITAL ARTERY PERFUSION

Brian R. Younge, M.D.

Recent literature has described little in the way of successful treatment of central retinal artery occlusion. However, since Rosenbaum's and my last communication in 1978 (1), I have had occasion to use the technique described by Watson (2) to treat eight more patients with central retinal artery occlusion.

CLINICAL ASPECTS

Patients presenting with or having an episode of acute loss of vision while at the Mayo Clinic usually are seen by a physician within a few minutes. If a central retinal arterial occlusion is diagnosed, the patient is considered to be a candidate for surgical intervention if the loss of vision occurred less than 24 hours from the time it was first noticed.

During the assessment of the patient, preparations are made for immediate transfer to the operating room. The patient may then be treated by conservative measures and, if these are unsuccessful, cannulation under local anesthesia may be carried out within an hour after diagnosis. This requires adequate preparation beforehand and rapid response of the operating room team. There is no time to prepare the patient for general anesthesia and no time for a carotid system work-up. There is only enough time to explain to the patient the desperate situation and the grim prognosis. Time is of the essence, the risks for permanent visual loss are very high, and only rapid restoration of circulation will permit recovery of vision.

After the situation is explained to the patient and relatives, an attempt should be made to cannulate and flush out the ophthalmic system. The idea

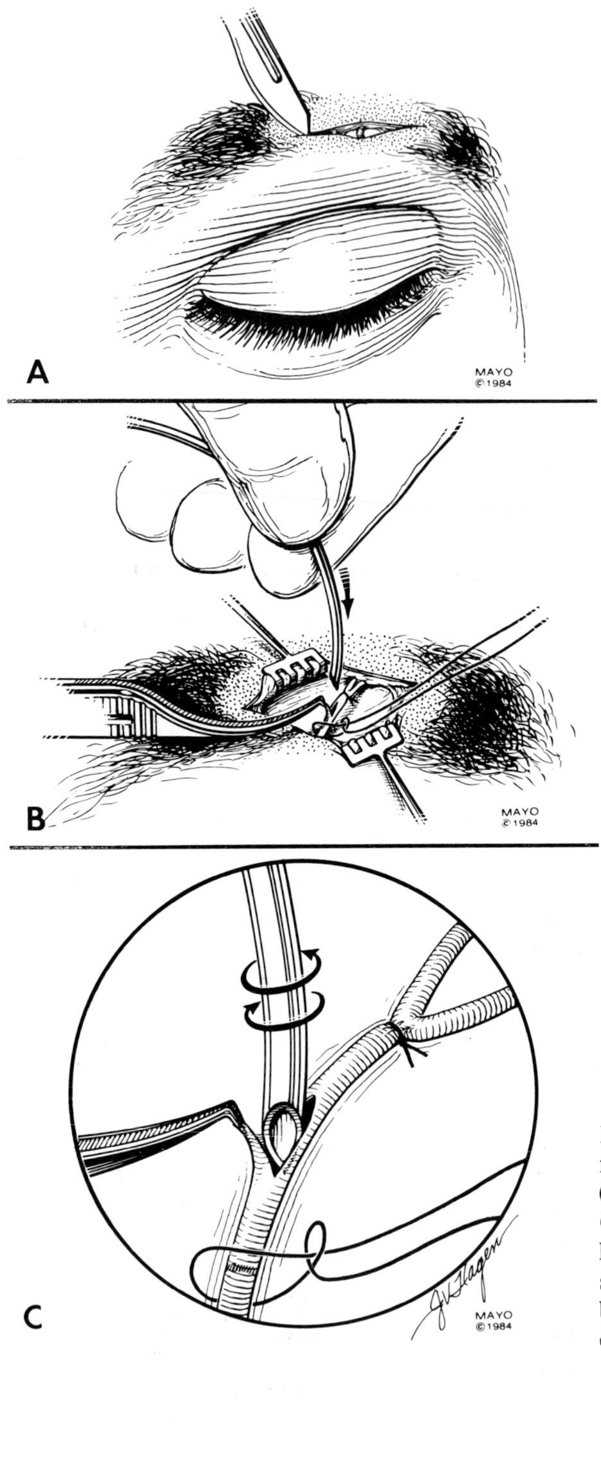

Fig. 16.1. Introduction of fine polyethylene catheter (PE 50/S36, Clay Adams Co.) into the supraorbital lumen. The vessel will be in spasm and so will appear bloodless. (By permission of Mayo Foundation.)

is to get substances to the area of blockage (at the lamina cribrosa or more proximally in the central retinal artery) in the hopes of inducing vasodilation and thrombolysis.

The total or almost total arrest of retinal circulation can be confirmed by the ophthalmoscopic appearance; retinal artery pressures must then be measured. The usual finding is total occlusion of the artery with segmentation (the so-called box car formation) of the venous return and a whitish opacity of the retina in the macula (cherry-red spot). If normal-appearing vessels are present with a normal retinal artery pressure but the patient has no vision, one should proceed no further. Retinal infarction is complete and any recovery will be unrelated to treatment. Emboli should be noted if present, and the carotid arteries should be auscultated for bruits.

METHODS

An anesthesiologist should be in attendance if available. Local anesthesia is induced, the supraorbital notch is palpated, and an incision is made over the notch to find the artery. It is important to realize that the vessel will be in spasm and may be difficult to distinguish from nerves in the same region. A small catheter usually can be passed into the lumen by using a twisting motion to get the beveled tip into the cut vessel (Figure 16.1). Upon injection of heparinized saline and papaverine, the vessel fills with arterialized blood which can be seen pulsing up into the cannula. Several injections of saline followed by papaverine are used to attempt to clear the central retinal artery.

If vision begins to return, the patient may be able to indicate an improvement in response to inquiry. Observation of the retina with the indirect ophthalmoscope and a cobalt filter after intraarterial injection of fluorescein will demonstrate circulation within the orbital tissues and, one hopes, in the central retinal artery. Even in the absence of this latter finding, a few patients will have recovered their vision to some extent by the next day. We have not used the Harvard infusion pump to date but plan to do so in the future, with the use of other agents.

RESULTS OF TREATMENT

Of the eight patients treated by supraorbital artery cannulation and retrograde perfusion with heparinized saline, papaverine, and lidocaine, three had recovery of vision—one to normal acuity and two to decreased but measurable vision (Table 16.1). The interval between loss of vision and treatment ranged from 6 to 18 hours. The best result occurred in a patient treated within 8 hours. Several of these patients were elderly, and several

TABLE 16.1. Effect of treatment on central retinal occlusions

Case	*Age (yrs)*	*Vision** *Preop.*	*Postop.*	*Time elapsed before treatment (hr)*	*Comment*
1	78	NLP	NLP	12	Died 2 years later, stroke
2	84	LP	LP	7	Carotid occluded distal to ophthalmic artery
3	46	NLP	NLP	6	Transient paresis, nerve III; later bypassed
4	75	CF	6/200	14	Embolus on disc moved
5	55	CF	20/25	8	Residual field defect
6	49	LP	LP	18	One eye blind already, vascular disease
7	63	HM	HM	16	Cherry-red spot unchanged
8	76	NLP	2/200	12	Retinal artery pressures; later normal

*HM, hand movements; NLP, no light perception; LP, light perception; CF, count fingers.

had significant medical, particularly vascular, problems. One has since died from a cerebrovascular accident, about a year after his episode of vision loss. Only one patient had a complication from the procedure, a partial paresis of cranial nerve III. This was of little consequence because the patient's paresis resolved; unfortunately his vision did not return.

The results of treatment by cannulation in these additional eight patients have been somewhat disappointing but nevertheless better than those of the usual approach. Newer techniques now used in treatment of coronary artery embolism, such as perfusion with streptokinase and some of the new thrombolytic agents, may improve these results in the future.

DISCUSSION

Even with no treatment, some patients recover vision spontaneously after retinal ischemia. Nonetheless, in few patients is flow reestablished in a sufficiently short time for the retina to recover function. Evidence from animal experiments suggests that total blockage of the central retinal arterial flow for several hours results in irreparable damage to the inner layers of the retina (3). Human retina probably has a similar time limit, but a definite value has not been established. I have witnessed recovery of flow within 24 hours after occlusion, with normalization of retinal arterial pressures but no return of vision. It seems hopeless, therefore, to undertake any sort of treatment in such a case and certainly hopeless if the circulation is still arrested. Recovery may depend upon the degree of occlusion, because a minor amount of flow may preclude vision yet be reversible after several hours or even a day. Judgment must be exercised in deciding which cases to undertake when occlusion has persisted for longer than 24 hours.

I plan to make use of streptokinase and other thrombolytic agents as they become available. Our cardiology colleagues have been successful in opening coronary arteries by direct infusion of streptokinase through a catheter introduced into the coronary artery ostium. Whether retrograde perfusion of the ophthalmic artery will deliver sufficient quantities of drug to the target embolus remains to be seen. In order to keep the quantity of streptokinase well below systemically fibrinolytic levels (over 100,000 units), I intend to use the following regimen for future suitable cases:

1 vial of streptokinase (250,000 units)
Saline, 18 ml
Nitroglycerin, 2 ml (80 μg/ml)

Mix the above in a 30-ml syringe (12,500 units/ml)
Place syringe in Harvard pump
Infuse at 12,500 units/min, i.e, 1.0 ml/min
Maximum dose, 7 ml (87,500 units)
Stop the infusion at half the maximum dose and
examine the fundus
Wait 15 minutes, reexamine the fundus
for evidence of improved blood flow,
and continue the infusion until the entire
7 ml has been given

This regimen should deliver adequate streptokinase to the ophthalmic system, and hopefully to the blocked central retinal artery, without producing systemic fibrinolysis or cerebral complications. The rate of infusion in the coronary arteries is half of the above rate, but the catheter is placed right next to the thrombus or at least into the ostium; whereas, in the supraorbital artery cannulation procedure, there is considerable retrograde distance and pressure to overcome and much of the drug will be lost in the other branches of the ophthalmic artery.

If the procedure is successful in restoring circulation, the patient should be heparinized for several days to prevent recurrence of thrombosis. He or she should also be treated with antiplatelet agents such as aspirin, 325 mg three times a day, and dipyridamole (Persantine), 75 mg three times a day (4). Because of their rather high incidence of carotid and other vascular diseases, including coronary artery disease, these patients should be evaluated carefully in the postoperative period. Because of the antibody-antigen reaction possible in repeat therapy, streptokinase should be administered only once and only if the patient has not been exposed to streptokinase previously.

It may take another few years to accumulate enough cases at the Mayo Clinic to provide sufficient data for a longer article on this technique. Because of the simplicity of the operation, the low risks, and the usual outcome of untreated central retinal artery occlusion, it seems reasonable to undertake this study, even in the absence of controls. As newer agents, such as tissue plasminogen activator (t-PA), become available which are more clot specific, don't cause systemic fibrinolysis, and are nonallergenic, the cannulation procedure may become more useful.

ACKNOWLEDGMENTS

The author thanks Dr. Hugh C. Smith of the Division of Cardiovascular Diseases and Internal Medicine at the Mayo Clinic for his advice on streptokinase infusions.

REFERENCES

1. Younge, B.R., Rosenbaum, T.J.: Treatment of acute central retinal artery occlusion. *Mayo Clin. Proc.* 53:408, 1978.
2. Watson, P.G.: The treatment of acute retinal arterial occlusion. In Cant, J.S., ed. *The William Mackenzie Centenary Symposium on the Ocular Circulation in Health and Disease*, London: Henry Kimptom, 1969, pp. 243-245.
3. Hayreh, S.S., Weingeist, T.A.: Experimental occlusion of the central artery of the retina. IV: Retinal tolerance time to acute ischaemia. *Brit. J. Ophthalmol.* 64:818, 1980.
4. Chesebro, J.H., Clements, I.P., Fuster, V., et al: A platelet-inhibitor-drug trial in coronary-artery bypass operations: Benefit of perioperative dipyridamole and aspirin therapy on early post-operative vein-graft patency. *N. Engl. J. Med.* 307:37, 1982.

17

TREATMENT OF CAROTID-CAVERNOUS FISTULAS WITH DETACHABLE BALLOONS

Alfredo Lazo, M.D.

The carotid-cavernous fistula is produced by rupture of the wall of the internal carotid artery, or one of its branches, into the cavernous sinus. After the rupture, blood flows under high pressure into the dural cavernous sinus (1). The etiology of the fistula in more than two thirds of the patients is head trauma (2,3). Other causes are ruptured cavernous carotid aneurysm and iatrogenic problems following transphenoidal surgery (4).

ANATOMY AND ANGIOGRAPHY

The rent of a carotid-cavernous fistula is most commonly located in the horizontal intracavernous portion of the internal carotid artery. The fistula varies in size from 1 to 5 mm with an average size of 3 mm. In the majority of the patients there is only one rent but two have been described (2).

The affected carotid artery may enlarge as the result of increased blood flow. Distal to the fistula, the blood flow may be diminished (Figure 17.1 A,B). Rarely, there is a total steal, with all the carotid blood flow draining into the fistula. In these patients the anterior and middle cerebral arteries on the affected side are filled through the anterior or posterior communicating arteries. The external carotid artery does not contribute to the fistula in most patients.

The venous drainage is related to the location of the fistula. If anteriorly located, the drainage is initially through the superior ophthalmic vein. Subsequent flow is through the angular, facial and external jugular vein. The posterior drainage is through the inferior and superior petrosal sinuses. Concominant flow exists between the posterior and anterior

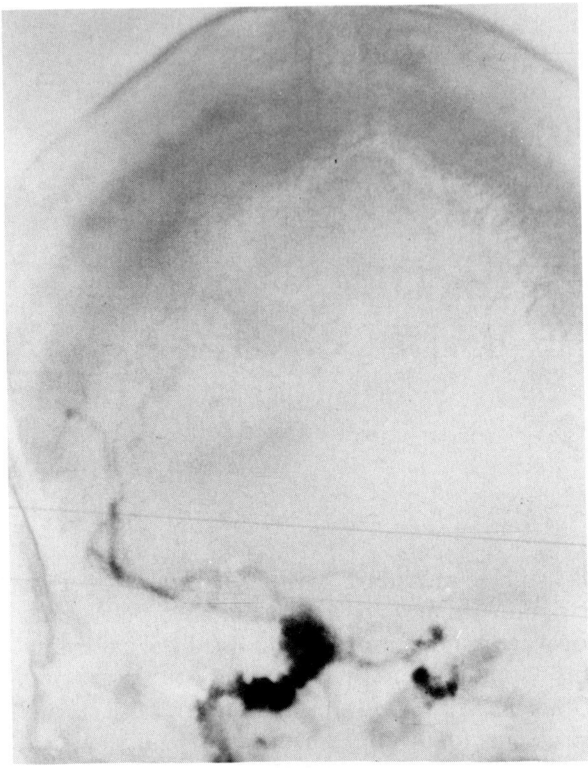

Fig. 17.1. Right internal carotid arteriogram showing a carotid-cavernous fistula. There is poor filling of the right middle cerebral artery.

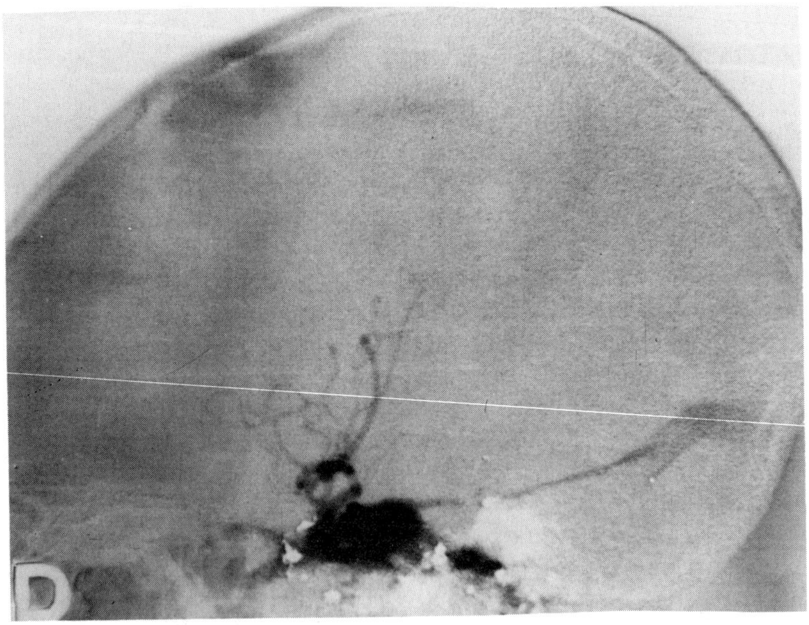

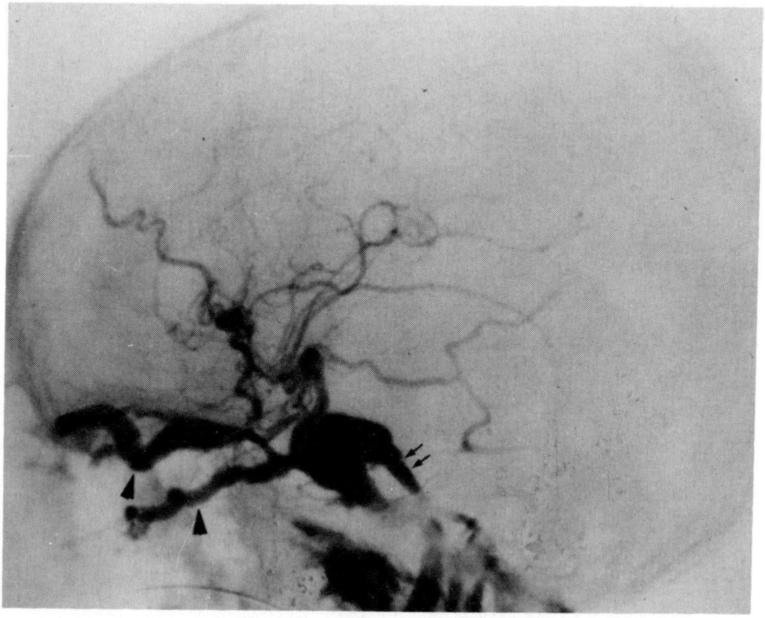

Fig. 17.2. Large carotid-carvernous fistula with superior ophthalmic vein (*arrow heads*) and inferior petrosal sinus drainage (*arrows*). Notice the occlusion of posterior branches of the right middle cerebral artery.

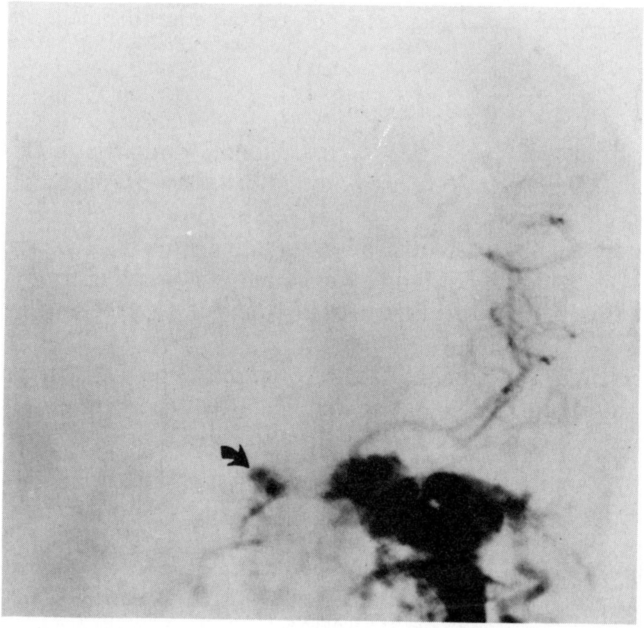

Fig. 17.3. Left carotid-cavernous fistula with contra-lateral drainage (*arrow*).

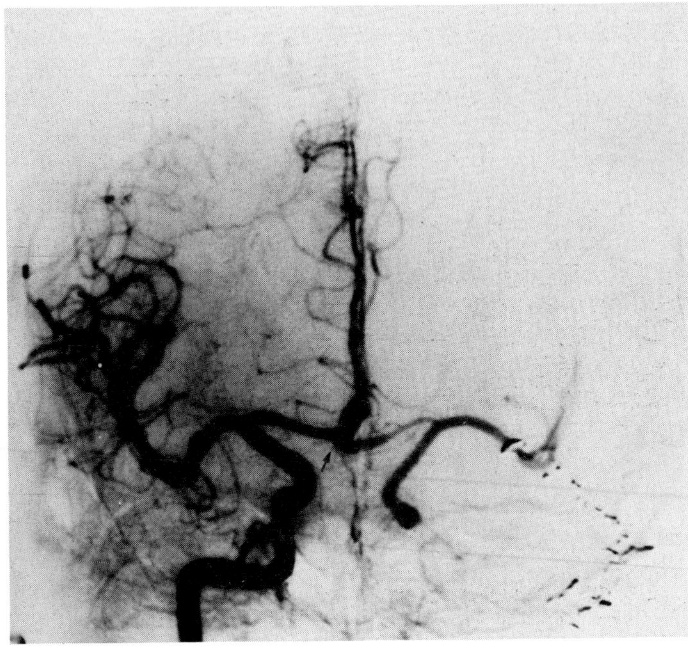

Fig. 17.4. Right internal carotid arteriogram with compression of the left common carotid artery demonstrating patency of the anterior communicating artery (*arrow*).

drainage systems (Figure 17.2). Contralateral drainage is through the coronal veins (Figure 17.3). This flow pattern may produce contralateral proptosis and chemosis.

The angiographic demonstration of the fistula is accomplished by conventional carotid angiography with rapid film imaging techniques. The purpose of this preembolization arteriography is to precisely localize the fistula site.

It is essential to visualize both the vertebral-basilar system and the internal carotid arteries angiographically. The vertebral arteriogram is performed with compression of the affected carotid artery to demonstrate the patency of the posterior communicating artery. The normal internal carotid artery is injected while the opposite carotid artery is being compressed to show cross filling through the anterior communicating artery (Figure 17.4). If such communications exist, sacrificing the internal carotid artery may be possible without serious neurological consequences.

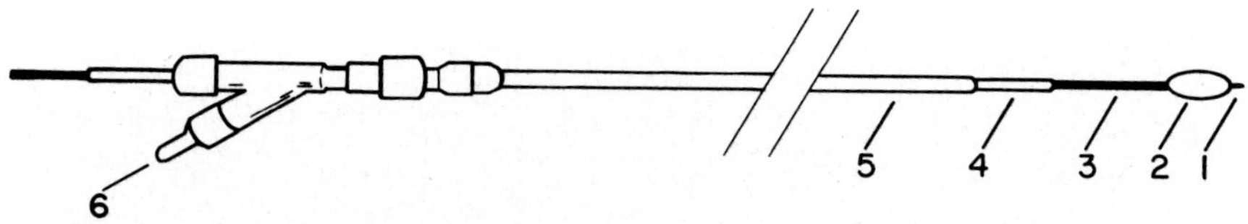

Fig. 17.5. Detachable balloon catheter system: 1, metallic clip; 2, balloon; 3, balloon catheter; 4, detaching catheter; 5, introducing catheter; 6, side arm for heparinized saline solution.

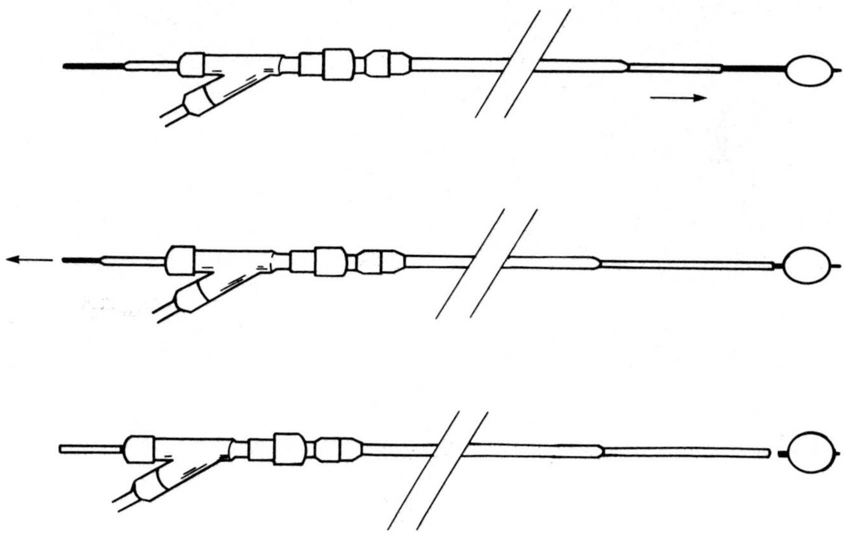

Fig. 17.6. Balloon detachment (top to bottom): 1, detaching catheter is advanced to the neck of the balloon; 2, balloon catheter is pulled to detach the balloon; 3, balloon is detached.

CLINICAL FINDINGS

The carotid-cavernous fistulas are almost invariably traumatic in origin. The symptoms are usually unilateral, and are related to the increased pressure in the veins that normally drain the orbit (1).

These patients present clinically with pulsating exophthalmos with pain, engorgement of the conjunctival and retinal vessels and disturbances of external ocular movements (4). Blurred vision and loud bruit in the

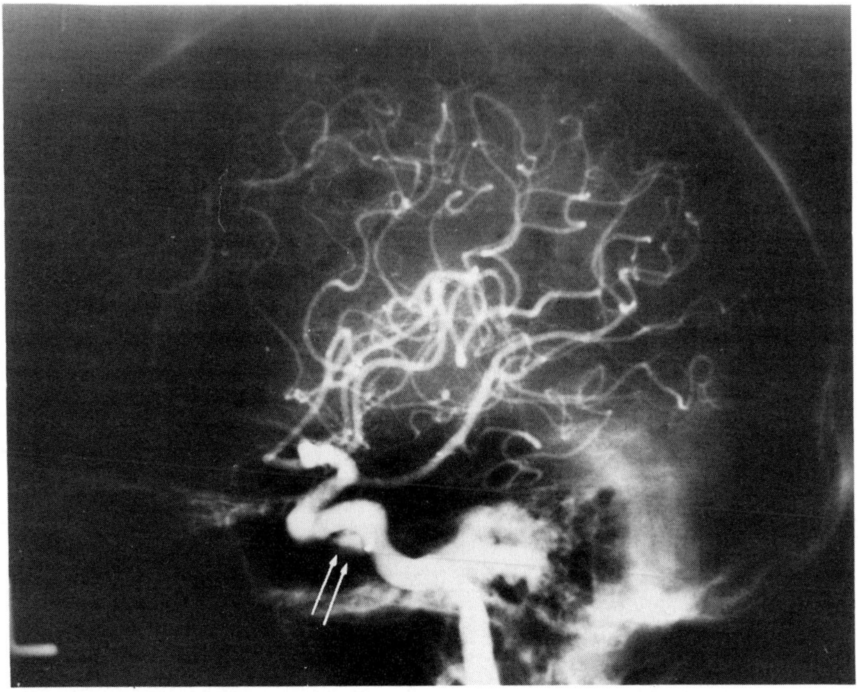

Fig. 17.7. Left internal carotid arteriogram following balloon embolization (*arrows*). There is complete occlusion of the carotid-cavernous fistula. The internal carotid has a normal diameter.

orbital region may also be noted. The third, fourth, and sixth cranial nerves may be affected by the fistula.

The symptoms usually begin within 24 hours following the development of the fistula, but occasionally they appear weeks later.

TREATMENT

The carotid-cavernous fistula is not a life-threatening condition. The importance of an early treatment is to preserve or improve vision, return the orbit and its content to normal and to eliminate the bruit (5).

Multiple surgical procedures have been used to treat cavernous-carotid fistulas, most requiring sacrifice of the internal carotid artery. The intravascular approach started with Brooks (6) in 1930 with the use of small pieces of muscle to embolize the fistula. Fogarty catheters had previously been utilized for permanent occlusion of this lesion.

Newer and more sophisticated techniques include the development of detachable balloons made of latex or silastic (2, 7–12). Kerber (13) designed a calibrated leak balloon catheter which, in conjunction with bucrylate, successfully sealed a carotid-cavernous fistula.

The percutaneous interventional method described in this presentation was developed by Servinenko (11) in 1974 and perfected by Debrun et al. (2, 8). This technique involves the percutaneous (transfemoral or direct common carotid approach) insertion of a large 7-8F catheter into the internal carotid artery (Figure 17.5). This catheter is connected to a Y adapter. The side arm of this adapter is constantly perfused with heparinized saline solution. The direct end of the Y connector is utilized for the introduction of the balloon catheter. This catheter is a 2F Teflon flexible tube that has a latex balloon tied to the end with latex threads. A small silver clip within the balloon tip permits fluoroscopic visualization and positioning. The balloon catheter is introduced together with a 3F sheath catheter as a coaxial system. Following proper positioning of the balloon within the carotid-cavernous fistula, the balloon is inflated by injecting an isotonic solution of metrizamide (170 mg/cc) (14). An arteriogram may then be performed to determine if there is complete occlusion of the fistula. If necessary, the position or size of the balloon may be modified.

In order to detach the balloon (Figure 17.6), the 3F sheath catheter is advanced until it is in contact with the base of the balloon. The inner catheter is then pulled backwards, enabling detachment of the balloon. The latex threads act as valve thus preventing deflation (Figure 17.7).

The size of the balloon will gradually diminish and within a month's time will be totally deflated (2). This time period is sufficient to produce thrombosis of the fistula. A silicone mixture may be substituted for the metrizamide and will harden within the balloon in 10 to 15 minutes. One of the problems arising from the utilization of the silicone mixture is the dead space within the catheters which makes total replacement of the metrizamide impossible. New double lumen catheters are being developed that will solve this problem.

In some cases because of the location of the rent, the balloon cannot be positioned within the fistula. In these patients, the internal carotid artery may be occluded with one balloon at the opening of the fistula or with two balloons, one proximal and one distal to the rent (figure 17.8 A, B). This procedure can be performed only if the anterior or posterior communicating arteries are patent, and the patient's clinical condition does not deteriorate subsequent to balloon inflation.

A transfemoral or transjugular venous approach to the cavernous-carotid fistula can be used when the main venous drainage is through the inferior petrosal sinus and jugular vein (2, 15). The risk of cerebral embolization diminishes when the venous route is used.

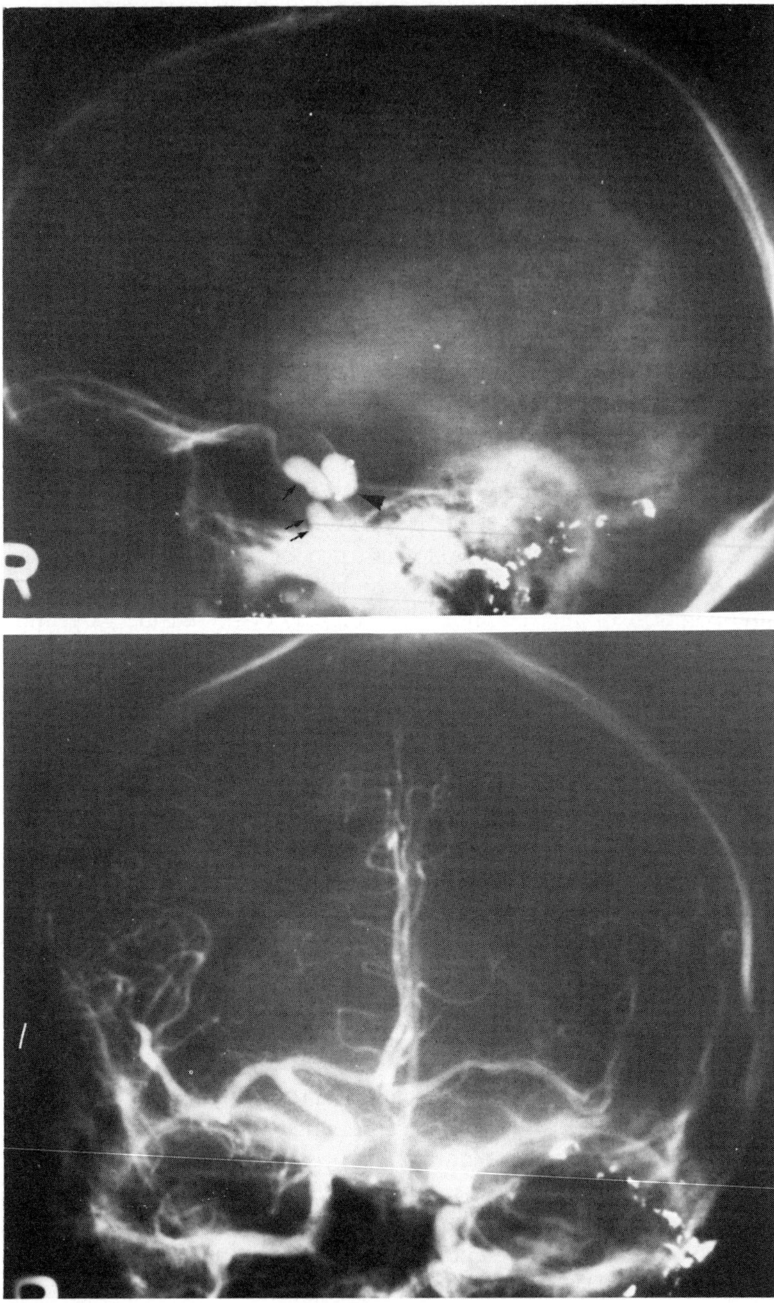

Fig. 17.8. Carotid-cavernous fistula in a 40-year-old patient following self-inflicted bullet wound. **a:** First balloon (*arrow head*) did not occlude the carotid-cavernous fistula. The internal carotid was then occluded with two balloons, one proximal (*arrow*) and one distal (*two arrows*) to the rent. **b**: Right internal carotid arteriogram following embolization shows filling of the left middle cerebral artery through the anterior communicating artery.

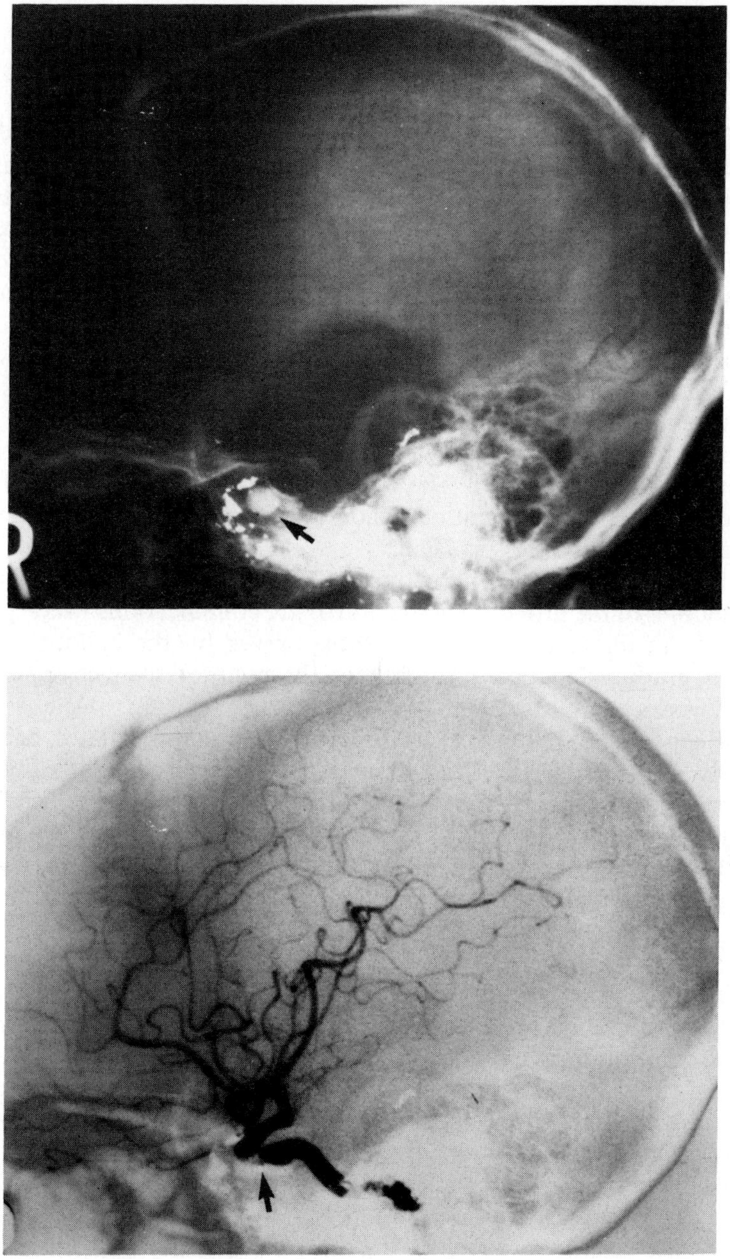

Fig. 17.9. Carotid-cavernous fistula following gunshot wound to the right petrous bone. **a:** Lateral view following detachment of the balloon into the carotid-cavernous fistula (*arrow*). **b:** Right internal carotid arteriogram demonstrating narrowing of the internal carotid artery at the balloon site (*arrow*). There is good filling of the right anterior and middle cerebral arteries.

COMPLICATIONS

The treatment of carotid-cavernous fistulas with detachable balloons is not without risk. One of the problems encountered with this technique is hematoma at the puncture site. The risk of this complication is greater when a direct carotid puncture is performed rather than the conventional percutaneous transfemoral method of insertion. A prolonged period of pressure should be applied to the site of puncture. If systemic heparinization is used during the embolization, its anticoagulative effect may have to be reversed with protamine sulfate (5). Symptomatic false aneurysms (2) are formed when the balloon deflates rapidly, usually as the result of a defective ligature. The distal part of the fistula is thrombosed, but the proximal part remains as a cavity connected with the carotid artery. A false aneurysm is then created. The symptoms include pain and oculomotor nerve palsy. The permanent occlusion of the internal carotid artery with a balloon will resolve this problem.

Isolated oculomotor nerve palsy (2, 5) and facial pain related to the distribution of the fifth cranial nerve (10) are complications which probably result from direct pressure upon these nerves by the balloon. With the normal gradual deflation of the balloon the symptoms will disappear within a few weeks.

Reopening of the fistula may occur if the balloon deflates, or migrates distally before the fistula is completely thrombosed. Clinically all the symptoms will reappear. The ideal treatment is to occlude the fistula with a second balloon. If this is not possible, the internal carotid artery may have to be occluded with balloons. Rupture of the balloon can be avoided with proper selection of size in relationship to the fistula. The volume of contrast used for inflation should not be excessive.

Systemic heparinization during the procedure is recommended to eliminate the possibility of thrombus formation within the catheter. Such clot formation may propagate distally into the cerebral circulation.

Protrusion of the balloon out of the fistula and into the lumen of the internal carotid artery sometimes occurs (Figure 17.9 A,B). Although flow through the narrowed segment of the internal carotid artery still is noted, emboli may form and seed distally into the cerebral arteries. Systemic heparinization may be considered in such cases.

REFERENCES

1. Newton, T.H., Potts, D.G.: *Radiology of the skull and brain.* St. Louis: C.V. Mosby, 1974.
2. Debrun, G., Lacour, P., Vinuela, F., Fox, A., Drake, C.G., and Caron, J.P.: Treatment of fifty-four traumatic carotid cavernous fistulas. *J. Neurosurg.* 55:678, 1981.

3. Taveras, J.M., Wood, E.H.: *Diagnostic Neuroradiology*. Baltimore: Williams and Wilkins, 1976.
4. Mumenthauler, M.: *Neurology*. Year Book Medical Publishers, Inc. George Thieme, 1977.
5. Barrow, D.L., Fleischner, A.S., and Hoffman, J.C.: Complications of detachable balloon catheter technique in the treatment of traumatic intracranial arteriovenous fistulas. *J. Neurosurg.* 56:396, 1982.
6. Brooks, B.: The treatment of traumatic arteriovenous fistula. *South. Med. J.* 23:100, 1930.
7. Berenstien, A., Kricheff, I.I.: Catheter and material selection for transarterial embolization: technical considerations. *Radiology* 132:619, 1979.
8. Debrun, G., Lacour, P., Caron, J.P., et al: Experimental approach to the treatment of carotid cavernous fistulas with an inflatable and isolated balloon. *Neuroradiology* 9:9, 1975.
9. Fierstien, S.B., DeFeo, D., and Nutkiewicz, A.: Complete obliteration of a carotid fistula with sparing of the carotid blood flow using a detachable balloon catheter. *Surg. Neurol.* 9:277, 1978.
10. Norman, D., Newton, T.H., Edwards, M.S. and DeCaprio, V.: Carotid cavernous fistula: closure with detachable silicone balloons. Radiology 149:149, 1983.
11. Serbinenko, F.A.: Balloon catheterization and occlusion of major cerebral vessels. *J. Neurosurg.* 41:125, 1974.
12. White, R.I., Kaufman, S.L., Barth, K.H., DeCaprio, V., and Strandbert, J.D.: Embolotherapy with detachable silicone balloons. *Radiology* 131:619, 1979.
13. Kerber, C.W., Bank, W.O., Cromwell, L.D.: Cyanoacrylate occlusion of carotid cavernous fistula with preservation of carotid artery flow. *Neurosurgery* 40:110, 1974.
14. Barth, K.H., White, R.I., Kaufman, S.L., and Strandberg, J.D.: Metrizamide, the ideal radiopaque filling material for detachable silicone balloon embolization. *Invest. Radiol.* 14:35, 1979.
15. Manelfe, C., Berenstien, A.: Treatment of carotid cavernous fistulas by venous approach. *J. Neuroradiol.* 7:13, 1980.

DISCUSSION: SESSION THREE

RELATIONSHIP BETWEEN ION AND CAROTID ARTERY DISEASE

A substantial part of the material presented at the meeting attempted to define the relationship between ischemic optic neuropathy (ION) and carotid artery disease. Some patients develop ION as a complication of giant cell arteritis. In the majority, however, an arteritis cannot be proven. In this latter group carotid disease is prevalent and the ischemia of the head of the optic nerve may be due to hypoperfusion from stenosis of the carotid or ophthalmic arteries, microemboli passing from atheromatous lesions in the carotid artery to the posterior ciliary arteries or so-called "small vessel disease" of the short posterior ciliary arteries. In what percentage of patients carotid disease is merely coincidental is not known. Of those patients whose carotid disease is presumed to be the cause of ION, it is impossible to define with reasonable certainty which ones are due to microemboli and which to hypoperfusion.

This relationship between atheroma of the carotid bifurcation and ION prompted many practical questions dealing with the management of patients with ION.

IS STANDARD ARTERIOGRAPHY INDICATED IN PATIENTS WITH ION?

Should all patients with ION have a carotid arteriogram as an emergency procedure? Weiss stressed that most of the patients that were being discussed had either CRAO or ION. Those patients with CRAO should have an arteriogram, if not as an emergency, certainly in an expedient manner. He was not sure which patients with ION should have an arteriogram. Intravenous digital arteriography does not have enough resolution to properly evaluate the carotid arteries in these patients. Weiss stated that a certain number of patients will turn out to have microembolization to the posterior ciliary arteries, but he did not know the incidence of this mechanism in the total group of patients with ION.

Russell did not recommend arteriography for patients with ION. Although he agreed with the advisability of doing ultrasound, he believes ION is primarily "small vessel disease" and hence factors such as hypertension, smoking, and others traditionally linked with small vessel disease should be investigated.

Magargal suggested excluding first those patients with ION of the arteritic type; these patients need steroids and, he feels, there is no point in doing an arteriogram in them. He stated that if he saw a patient with ION of the nonarteritic type who had no other signs of carotid disease (which he defined as absence of bruits, good pulses, and no history of transient ischemic attacks), he would not do an arteriogram. He believes that in these patients, the most important underlying systemic factor is hypertension rather than carotid disease. In other words, he would only do an arteriogram if the patient had a bruit or some other clinical evidence of carotid disease.

Clearly, Magargal's definition of *absence of carotid disease* will miss many patients with small, subcritical atheromata with ulceration and surface thrombi quite capable of producing embolization of the orbital arterial supply.

Weiss felt that all these patients should have thorough noninvasive testing and imaging. If the noninvasive exam suggests a carotid lesion, an arteriogram is indicated. He also pointed out that ION often develops later in the opposite eye (40% of nonarteritic type). Therefore, in patients with ION in whom temporal arteritis has been ruled out, one should be aware that the other eye is at significant statistical risk for developing ION. The ION may be secondary to embolization, so this is another reason to do noninvasive testing and again, if results are positive, proceed with an arteriogram.

The group agreed that no evidence supports the prescription of an arteriogram as an emergency procedure in a patient with ION. In some patients, however, elective arteriography will reveal a carotid lesion which is not only the possible etiology of the ION, but also presents a risk for stroke.

In view of the facts and new findings presented there was consensus that it is time to initiate a prospective study to ascertain the relationship between ION and carotid artery disease.

HENKIND'S MODEL

After Henkind's presentation, the question arose as to why more of the experimental animals did not show evidence of venous stasis retinopathy or so-called ocular hypoperfusion syndrome. Henkind responded that during the course of their follow-up, a number of the experimental animals developed cataracts, presumably as a result of anterior segment ischemia. These animals were eliminated from the study because follow-up fluorescein angiograms could not be performed on them, a requirement of the experimental protocol. He indicated that in future studies he would look very carefully at these animals that develop cataracts. Perhaps these are the ones that will demonstrate evidence of the so-called venous stasis retinopathy (ocular hypoperfusion).

Young pointed out that the retinal changes seen in hypoperfusion retinopathy occur in ischemic but not in infarcted retinas. Probably the acute circulatory arrest produced in Henkind's experimental model precludes these characteristic findings of ocular hypoperfusion. He suggested that prolonged ischemia, rather than infarction, may be the condition causing development of the characteristic retinal vascular findings, just as it is in diabetes mellitus.

Henkind also mentioned some unusual electron-microscopic findings in the retina following experimental carotid artery occlusion. What he found, quite unexpectedly, were changes in the photoreceptors, especially at 16 weeks following occlusion. Henkind pointed out that his model certainly is not an exact duplication of a human situation; nevertheless it may provide us with important information.

He was asked why he considered the changes in the retinal capillary bed "protective" (referring to his findings of a focal drop-out of portions of the capillary bed). Henkind said that he had done other embolization experiments on the retinal vasculature, but he had never seen a picture quite like the one he achieved with this experiment. He interpreted the picture as one where there is limited drop-out of portions of the capillary bed in an effort to preserve the remaining capillary bed. In Henkind's model, individual capillary strands disappear within larger areas of intact capillary bed.

Finally, Henkind also pointed out another unusual finding in the retinal capillary bed: intramural pericytes increasing in number. This was the only situation he knew of where pericytes actually increased in number.

Henkind was asked why he found sheathing in the fundus of his experimental animals since he was doing carotid occlusions as opposed to embolization. He stated that it is possible to have embolization distal to a carotid occlusion, and this is a phenomenon that can be seen frequently in patients with carotid artery thrombosis propagating through the intracranial segment, fragmenting, and embolizing distally.

CARDIOVASCULAR PROGNOSIS OF PATIENTS WITH ION

The question was raised as to whether the prognosis of patients with ION is different from those with retinal stroke. Patients who have a retinal stroke caused by an embolus have a different lifespan and cardiovascular future than people who present with ION. Further, ION may not be an embolic complication from atheroma, and this might be why, in terms of myocardial infarction, the prognosis of these patients is different.

Berguer stated that the discussion of cardiovascular risk in this group should be limited to that majority of patients with ION labeled as idiopathic, the etiology of which is either embolism or hypoperfusion, probably from severe carotid disease. If one lumps all patients with ION in a single group, by including among them the patients whose ION is secondary to temporal arteritis, the risk characteristics of the group may change substantially.

A member of the audience stated that of all patients with ION, those whose disease is secondary to temporal arteritis represent perhaps 10%. The remaining majority is called idiopathic and these patients do not generally go on to have embolic complications in other territories. He quoted Schatz's work showing different life expectancies for patients with embolic disease of the retina and for those with ION. Hayreh mentioned that for the last ten years he has been studying prospectively the natural history of the disease, and he has had personal experience with more than 500 patients. About 20% of his patients had ION secondary to temporal arteritis. In the remaining 80% there was no evidence of arteritis. He stressed too the important differences between patients with ION and patients with occlusion of the CRA or of its branches.

IS HYPOPERFUSION THE MECHANISM OF ION?

In the latter group (occlusion of the CRA or of its branches) one can see the embolus in the majority of cases, and it is fair to assume that carotid embolization is the most common etiology. In anterior ION Hayreh felt that the etiology was usually hypoperfusion of the watershed zone rather than posterior ciliary arterial embolization. He related how these patients wake up in the morning and cannot see. He believes that their blood pressure falls during sleep, and the watershed zone becomes hypoperfused and ischemic during the night. When they wake up in the morning, they experience the results of such ischemia. Asked in how many of these patients the disease is secondary to straight carotid embolization, he did not know, but he felt it was a small proportion of them.

HYPERTENSION AND ION

The role of hypertension in these patients was also discussed and Hayreh, referring again to his personal series, thought that hypertension was much overplayed. In his view, the incidence of hypertension in these patients is no different than that which is found in the general population. He also felt that those patients who present with ION have a risk of dying of stroke or cardiac death similar to the general population.

FLUORESCEIN ANGIOGRAPHY IN ION

Hayreh proposed the use of fluorescein angiography to help select those patients with ION who should have carotid arteriography. He does fluorescein angiography in all patients with ION. For those patients who do not have temporal arteritis and show large choroidal filling defect or do not fill their posterior ciliary arteries at all, he recommends a carotid arteriogram. On the other hand, if the patient has just a small filling defect in the watershed zone, he does not recommend a carotid arteriogram because the yield for carotid lesions in these patients would be too small to justify the risk. Many of the panel felt that the diagnostic potential of noninvasive testing had not been fully exploited in Hayreh's series.

Hayreh was asked what he would do if presented with a 60-year-old patient with ION and no carotid bruit. Would he suggest an arteriogram? He said that he would first do a fluorescein angiogram: if the test indicated occlusion of one of the short ciliary processes of the posterior ciliary artery, he would recommend an arteriogram. If he found ischemia of the watershed zone he would not.

STANDARD ARTERIOGRAPHY IN ION

Berguer was asked why he advised a four-vessel study in these patients when a selective bilateral arteriogram would provide the same information. In other words, why add the risk of an arch injection and selective subclavian studies for visualization of the vertebrals? Berguer answered that in his experience, 60% of patients with ischemia of the retina or optic nerve head will show important carotid lesions. The four-vessel arteriogram provides the necessary information regarding not only the carotids but also the other vessels of the neck, and such information is needed when planning a carotid operation. He clarified that the visualization of the vertebral arteries is accomplished by injection into the subclavian artery rather than by selective catheterization of the vertebral origins which is both more difficult and riskier.

In Hasso's opinion, adding selective vertebral views increases the risk of the study but he agreed that one needs to do a complete four-vessel workup to properly diagnose occlusive disease of the neck vessels. In his hand a combination of digital and regular arteriographic techniques has worked best. He uses the intraarterial digital technique to obtain views of the aortic arch and its branches which permits the use of a small catheter and a small amount of dye. The same technique is used to display the carotid bifurcations and the origin of the vertebral arteries. For the intracranial views he recommends conventional arteriography. Thus, intraarterial digital techniques help to achieve a complete arteriographic evaluation at lesser risk.

Hasso also expressed great hopes for the use of nonionic contrast agents. He said that Metrizamide is now used in high-risk infants undergoing preoperative cardiac studies. He has been using metrizamide for external carotid injections and for spinal cord arteriography because this nonionic contrast medium causes less pain. He anticipated that new nonionic contrast agents will be on the market soon. In his view their only drawback is that they are more expensive than the standard iodine-based contrast agents.

EPIDEMIOLOGY OF ION

Dealing further with the subject of epidemiology Seikert warned that any specialist who receives selected patients may bias his estimation of the prevalence of the condition that he treats. He stated that perhaps half of the population over 50 years of age have some degree of atherosclerosis in one of the major cerebral arteries, either carotid or vertebral. Any statement as to the incidence of, for example, eye disease in this group of patients must be based on large epidemiological studies where findings may be compared with their incidence among the general population.

POSSIBLE MECHANISMS OF ION

Berguer was asked about his patients who presented with ischemic lesions of the retina and in whom he had shown disease of the origin of the ophthalmic artery. The questioner theorized that perhaps the ischemia was secondary to hypoperfusion rather than to an embolism, that is, related to the combination of a tandem lesion in the internal carotid artery and the ophthalmic artery takeoff. If the retinal circulation is autoregulated, the orbital hypoperfusion caused by the tandem lesion would affect the retinal much more than the choroidal side of the circulation. Berguer agreed that that was indeed a possibility.

POSSIBLE MECHANISMS OF ION

Hayreh was asked, if ION was mostly due to hypoperfusion, how was it that the commonest field defect was an altitudinal rather than a vertical one, not conforming to the vertical boundaries of the blood supply (watershed) he had shown in his fluorescein angiograms?

Hayreh had often pondered this question but he did not have the answer. He acknowledged that the upper half of the watershed shows filling defects much more often than the lower one. As to why this is, he could only speculate that perhaps gravity might be playing a part. He said that the superior temporal part of the disc is the commonest part involved in ischemia.

RETROGRADE PERFUSION OF SUPRAORBITAL ARTERY

The technique presented by Younge for retrograde cannulation of the supraorbital artery prompted questions from the audience regarding the safety of such a procedure. It might, in some cases, compromise an important source of collateral supply to the orbit, given the fact that the cannulated vessel is eventually ligated and becomes thrombosed. Younge did not think that the loss was important since there were other sources such as the nasociliary, lacrimal and other branches that contributed to the orbit in the same manner. In his view the loss of the supraorbital artery did not have the same importance as the sacrifice of a superficial temporal artery in a patient with internal carotid artery occlusion.

ARTERIOGRAPHY IN ION

Referring to the question of whether all patients who had ION should have an arteriogram or not, Berguer stressed that there are important differences between digital arteriography obtained by intravenous injection, regular arteriography, selective arteriography, and even superselective arteriography with high focus resolution or magnification techniques added. The latter techniques will show ophthalmic artery and posterior ciliary artery lesions that cannot be seen with intravenous or regular iodine contrast arteriography and can provide information on the mechanism of ischemia.

The preeminence of hypoperfusion—as opposed to microembolization—which Hayreh proposed as the etiology of ION, begs the suggestion that hypoperfusion of the orbit is also a reflection of the obstructive disease of the carotid and vertebral arteries causing orbital hypotension. This, in itself would justify doing an arteriogram (or at least noninvasive testing and imaging) to search for the obstructive lesion in the carotid bifurcation.

INDEX